Why Your Last Diet Failed You

And How This Book Won't Help You on Your Next One

by Charlie Hills

LOCK-SHIRE PRESS

Why Your Last Diet Failed You
And How This Book Won't Help You on Your Next One

Published by Lockshire Press
Printed in the United States of America
First Edition, October 2007

ISBN-10: 0-9749732-6-2
ISBN-13: 978-0-9749732-6-5

7 6 5 4 3 2 1

Disclaimer

As this book winds its way through a variety of stories and a range of moods, it's important to note that its primary purpose is simply to entertain. True, you'll get a fair share of opinion and commentary mixed in with the humor, but don't take it too seriously. I want you to have fun reading this.

I bring this up because weight control can be a sensitive subject. You're going to hear me whine like a spoiled baby about weight problems—*my* weight problems—which in all honest truth aren't much to get worked up over. I've never weighed four hundred pounds. I've never done anything remarkable or dramatic. I've never experienced a true life-threatening event. In short, I'm just whining.

I completely understand that someday someone weighing four hundred pounds might read this book. Someone with a much more remarkable story than mine is bound to read it and scoff at my moaning. The humor isn't intended to belittle or dismiss serious situations. It's to show that no matter how our individual issues stand up against each other, deep inside we're probably feeling pretty much the same. If that's the case, let's share a laugh or two. After all, next to Tylenol, laughter *is* the best medicine.

Contents

Preface

I'll level with you. This isn't going to be your usual diet book. If you've picked it up in the hopes of discovering the next big diet craze, then you may be disappointed. This is neither a diet revolution nor a doctor-designed, foolproof plan. I'm not a television star and I'm not hawking a barrage of related products. I'm a guy with a story. I've acquired (and re-acquired) a lot of pounds over the years and along with them, a lot of insight—into both myself and society at large.

The book's two goals are clearly spelled out in its title. I would like to help you understand why your last diet failed you. In a nutshell: it's not your fault. But I don't mean that in the usual, modern, lawsuit-laden, "everything is everybody else's fault" way of thinking. You'll see what I mean about that later.

Then, in what I believe is the most important message, I'll discuss how this book won't help you on your next diet. Now admittedly, it *might* help you. If you read it and learn something from it, there's a *chance* you could actually lose some weight. Unfortunately, the odds of that happening are stacked so high against you I must treat it as impossible.

"What? Why on earth would I read—or worse, *pay money for*—a diet book that tells me I have little or no hope of succeeding!?" Before you drop the book and run screaming to the nearest Dairy Queen, let me explain. Losing weight (and keeping it off) is hard work. There is simply no quick and easy way to do it. "Gee, now *there's* a real profound statement," you reply—and without the slightest hint of sarcasm. "You don't have to tell *me* that."

Well, to be perfectly honest, I think I *do* need to tell you that. Because when you look around at the typical sources of dieting help, you overwhelmingly find happy smiling people telling you how they lost 180 pounds in four days. They'll tell you how they ate anything they wanted, never had to exercise, and the pounds just melted away. Don't you see? You need the alternative viewpoint. You need a dose of reality. You need someone (and why not me?) to be the one to tell you in no uncertain terms, "This ain't gonna be easy."

But that's not what we want to hear, is it? Otherwise, why would we focus all our attention on the miracle diets? They tell us how easy it will be and we believe it. We believe it because we ache for it to be true. Though we know in our heart of hearts (or in our butt of butts) that hard work is the only true answer, we never stop believing that the Magic Pill is out there somewhere awaiting discovery. On that glorious day when we finally acquire it, we need only to swallow it and we'll be thin and beautiful again.

And we lived happily ever after.

Come on, people; wake up! Do you honestly believe this fairy tale will come true? Not likely. If you want to succeed, you simply must admit what you already know to be true: that losing weight and keeping it off for good means eating right and exercising.

There. I said it. Eat right and exercise.

But, oh if it were only that simple! Clearly it isn't, because if it were, the book would end right here. If it were, there wouldn't be tens of thousands of other books on the market all purporting to have The Answer. If it were, there wouldn't be happy, smiling people who'd lost 180 pounds in four days telling us their amazing stories on late night infomercials.

There's got to be more to it than just eating right and exercising. Otherwise, why do so few of us really give it a good, solid go? And why do even fewer of us succeed? And of those that actually do succeed, why is it that just a fraction keep it off permanently? Why can't we simply throw out the junk in our cupboards, replace it with healthful alternatives, walk a mile every morning, and just be done with it?

Why, why, why?

Well, if I answered all that in the Preface, I could probably only charge thirty-five cents for the book. As it stands, I have mortgage payments to make, so I'll pad it out a couple hundred more pages.

But I'll do more than pad. I'm going to tell you my story, and maybe—just maybe—you'll see some of your own story in these pages too. Maybe you'll come to understand more about why you've ended up where you have and why our society seems so nuts about this mammoth subject.

This book may be about dieting, but it's also supposed to be humorous. Additionally, if I've done my job right, you should find a few thought provoking ideas woven haphazardly amongst the funny bits. But most of all, I just want you to feel good after reading it—even if I can't help you on your next diet.

Why Your Last Diet Failed You

And How This Book Won't Help You on Your Next One

Chapter 1

Not Again

Darn it all. I did it again. And to be honest, I don't have any rational or logical explanation for it. The diet was going well. I started happily on Monday, kept it up Tuesday, still felt great on Wednesday, sailed through Thursday, and then last night we had pizza. Ahhh...pizza! Food of the gods. What mere mortal can exhibit any form of resistance in its powerful presence? The warm crispy crust, the tangy tomato sauce, the hot gooey cheese, and best of all, the sweating pepperoni. *Yum.* Who can resist? Not I, for one—a fact which has become excruciatingly obvious over the years.

So goes another five days of sacrificing down the drain. (Or down the esophagus, I should say.) And do you know what? I don't care. A week of denial is more than worth the five minutes of sweating pepperoni. At least that's what I tell myself during the heat of pizza passion. It's not until the next morning—yes, the proverbial "morning after"—that regret sets in. And guess what? Suddenly I *do* care. Those five minutes were *not* worth an entire week of sacrifice. But do you think that matters? Have I ever learned anything from it? Will the following Monday finally be my very last *Day One*?

If I know anything about myself, the answers to these three questions are *no*, *no*, and *no*.

Anyway, all philosophical questions aside, it's now Saturday morning and time to step on the scale again. Sure, I had one or two (or six) slices of pizza, but after losing three pounds over the previous week, it can't put *that* big a dent in the overall program, can it?

Ha! If you believe that then you are obviously not acquainted with *The Physical Laws of Dieting*. The first law states, "Weight returns at five times the velocity at which it was lost." The second law states, "Any dietary straying, no matter how seemingly insignificant, causes instantaneous Diet Reversal."

As it stands, I am very well acquainted with these laws (having made them up myself). And so it is this very knowledge that grants me foresight: I know exactly what will happen after I walk into the bathroom and step on that scale. These Laws cannot be broken. They cannot be bent. I am doomed. Yet I try to convince myself that *maybe just this once* I'll avoid the unavoidable. My mind reels, searching for facts and theories that might help me avert my impending doom. Then it hits me. "Traditional calorie theory!" my mind exclaims. "Yes, that will help me. I remember hearing something about how it takes an extra 3,500 calories to gain a pound." This is good. This is very good. I quickly begin doing some mental math. "Let's see, in order for me to gain back the three pounds I lost this week that implies I would have had to take in 10,500 extra calories last night. There's *no way* I ate *that* much pizza. No way."

Still, there's no sense taking any unnecessary chances. I head to the bathroom, pee, strip down, and jettison all unnecessary ballast, right down to my wedding ring. (Hey, every gram counts.) Here we go…

Unbelievable. I gained three pounds overnight. The Laws of Dieting win…*again*. I believe that brings the lifetime tally to *Laws*: 972, *me*: 0.

I say "unbelievable" but it really isn't. In fact, it's quite the opposite. It's very believable. (The previous 971 times kind of clued me into that.) As I step off the scale unsurprised, but nonetheless dejected, I briefly consider just giving up. But something always keeps me coming back. My desire for pizza, it would seem, is only equaled by my desire for punishment. The cycle continues.

This very scene, which I have personally played out over and over again, is one of the things that has led me to write this book. But it's not the only thing. I am nowhere near alone in my predicament. All you have to do is turn on the television or open a magazine or—or heck, all you have to do is just be alive. There's simply no escaping it. Weight loss—and our culture's obsession with it—is everywhere.

Worst of all, it doesn't seem like it's going away any time soon. No matter which diet is in vogue, or what new abdominal equipment is being peddled on late-night television, or even which Suzanne Somers book is currently at number one on Amazon.com, the problem *never goes away*.

I've watched this phenomenon for years, both on and off the playing field, and the longer I've watched, the more intrigued I've become. Most fascinating of all has been the fact that everyone and his uncle has come forth with a solution to the problem, yet no one seems to be getting any better. Not by any significant amounts.

But I'm getting ahead of myself. No one wants to hear the end of a story told before its beginning. (Well, no one except Star Wars fans.) So let's take a trip back in time and see how I got here.

Chapter 2

Scared Slim

The girth of my midsection went largely unnoticed (by me) for several years, despite its obvious, steady growth. Looking back now, I find this extraordinarily hard to believe. Not the fact that it was growing, but the fact that I hardly noticed it. I mean, I can't even imagine a time when I *wasn't* paying any attention to it, given my subsequent (and inordinate) preoccupation with the topic.

Then one fine spring morning in 1990, I clearly remember lying in bed looking down at my stomach. I stared at it a bit with an odd, sudden interest and thought *where on earth did that big, fat belly come from?* I puzzled about it for some time but try as I might, I simply couldn't figure it out. I had no recollection of ordering it from a catalog. I don't think I got it for Christmas. *Whence came you, O belly so great!?*

That's when I recalled one of my favorite quotes: "When you have eliminated the impossible, whatever remains, however improbable, must be the truth." That's it, of course! The only obvious explanation was that this big, fat belly had been delivered to the wrong address, because it sure as heck didn't belong to me. And now that I think about it, I'm sure it was supposed to go to that one guy, two apartments down on the other side of the hall. He always did look suspicious.

Anyway, after getting over the initial anger of this unjust affliction, I realized that, like it or not, it was now my burden and I had to do something about it. So I bought my very first bathroom scale. That's all. I just bought the scale. I didn't start a diet. I didn't jump up and go for a jog. I just wanted to begin collecting data. After all, I was single, 24, and had far better things to think about than weight control.

Then on May 7, 1990, I got my real first shocker. After about a week of weighing in around the mid 190s, I saw a horrible, horrible sight: the kind of vision that ends up burned into your memory forever. I looked down at the scale, and much to my dismay, it read *two zero zero point zero.* Two hundred? Two hundred! That just couldn't be right. I quickly stepped off and right back on again. Two hundred pounds. I mean, 195 seemed bad, but that was at least somewhat *manageable.* This—this was completely different. Two hundred pounds. I doubt I would have been any more surprised if it had said four hundred, or seven hundred, or even two thousand. I mean, this is the same guy who topped out at 145 in high school.

Two hundred pounds.

One might think that tipping the scales at one tenth of a ton would immediately force oneself into a strict diet program and/or exercise regimen. Surprisingly, I tried neither. Perhaps it was out of shock or maybe just out of sheer disbelief (if not outright denial). Either way, I did nothing about it, and only four days later was back down to the mid 190s. "Hmmm," I thought to myself. "It must have just been an anomaly."

For some odd reason, I continued to weigh myself and write it down almost daily. This went on for a few months until mid-August when just as quickly as I began, I quit. No more daily weigh-ins. I don't know exactly why I stopped. I can only assume I just got bored with it.

Boredom or not, intense interest in the subject abruptly returned on the morning of October 7, 1990. That's when I received my second shocker. This time the number *two zero five point zero* displayed as the scale glared at me. Oh yes, believe me, she* was most definitely glaring. This is what scales live for: the delivery of bad news. They delight in the telling. But on your peril, you must *not* give them the satisfaction. They are evil and must not be appeased. It only increases their power. Keep a poker face, quietly step off, and leave the room. It's our only hope against them.

So I did just that. I walked away, feeling rather numb. As I stumbled out of the bathroom, pondering this new large number, I wasn't quite certain what to think. Two hundred was bad, to be sure, but this was different. This was now *clearly* in the realm of the unimaginable. More than just a new high, I had squarely landed in a strange and unexplored territory. Welcome to the next level.

I must admit, it definitely had me somewhat scared. (No, not the type of scared where the doctor warns you to, "Lose weight or die." My situation was nothing so dramatic and I offer my apologies if you were hoping for something a bit more catastrophic based on the chapter title.)

I was mightily perturbed nonetheless and I will tell you one thing: this time I did not just sit back and watch. I definitely did something about it. Not knowing what else to do, I tried the craziest thing I could think of. I decided to eat better and start exercising. I know! Going out on the ol' limb there, wasn't I?

I tackled the issue of excess calories first. At the time, Slim Fast was riding a wave of popularity, so I figured: why not? For exercising, I decided to do something I hadn't done in a long time. I went swimming. It was a natural choice:

---

* Your scale is the opposite sex. I bet you didn't know that. (You'll think twice the next time you step on it naked, won't you?)

- I'd just joined a health club with a decent pool.
- I had to do something I wouldn't thoroughly hate.*
- I loved the smell of chlorine.

Not to mention I actually enjoyed it. In fact, I even swam a whole mile once. Back when I was around eleven or twelve, I went to a Boy Scout summer camp. Like all good camps, there was a lake nearby and the scouts had a special Mile Swim program. We called it "The Rocky Squad." (The movie had come out just a year or two before and the camp leaders apparently found themselves inspired by Mr. Balboa—not that I remembered Rocky swimming during his training.)

The lake was one half mile across. All each swimmer had to do was get to the other side and back. That's it. He was now a full-fledged member of the Rocky Squad. This didn't sound too bad so I decided to give it a go. On the morning of the event, my fellow challengers and I met up with the swim leader down by the lakeshore. We waded into the chilly water to the strains of *Gonna Fly Now* blaring from the camp PA system and began our watery trek.

It was a bit harder than I expected. I was continually forced to change strokes as various muscle groups wore out on me. Indeed, about halfway through, I was getting so worn out I decided I couldn't make it the whole way. So I turned around and swam back to the beginning.

Ha ha. Just kidding.

All told, it took me forty-five minutes to complete the trip, but I did it—and I'm not ashamed to admit I felt proud.

My warm, fuzzy feelings of self-accomplishment lasted until breakfast the next morning. Do you remember the part in the movie where Rocky begins his training by drinking all those raw eggs? Well, apparently one's membership in the Rocky Squad was only half-fledged until one performed a similar feat. Everyone who completed the swim the day before

---

* Can you say "treadmill"?

had to stand up in front of the entire mess hall and drink a raw egg. Juice glasses containing one fresh egg apiece were brought out on a tray and handed to each swimmer.

Oh no. I like my eggs over hard. *Very* hard, mind you. (Not to mention *hot*.) The tiniest bit of runny yoke makes me gag like a *Fear Factor* contestant wolfing down banana slugs. And suddenly I found myself in front of the entire camp, put on the spot by a silly tradition that had nothing to do with one's swimming prowess—expected to down an egg in the runniest format possible.

Putting my panic aside, I grasped my "juice" glass with firm resolve. Steely eyed, I stared down the barrel at the slimy bullet with my name on it. As the din around me rose, so too did the tension. But I had no choice. There was no turning back. I had to do this deed.

Within moments, at a countdown helpfully provided by two hundred shouting scouts, I tossed it back. Ugh. I can't imagine a banana slug being much worse than this. At least phase one was complete, though: I got it into my mouth. Then I made a small but profound tactical error. I held it at the back of my throat a bit too long (though definitely not on purpose). Ugh. My limited options flashed before me in an instant. Worried about the only other alternative, I summoned the nerve to swallow it. Phase two complete. I embarked upon the return journey to my seat, when after only a few short steps my stomach cried out, "What the hell is *this*?" and promptly returned the egg for a full refund.

The egg, nearly intact during flight, hit the ground with a sickening *splat*. The entire camp roared with laughter. Now it's natural to think I might have died of embarrassment right then and there, but to be honest, the whole thing was too darn funny. I laughed right along with everyone else. The swim leader caught up with me after breakfast. Wiping a tear from his eye, he said he'd never had *that* happen before. I should go back one day and see if there's a commemorative plaque on the mess hall wall sporting my name.

The Egg Incident certainly didn't put me off swimming forever. And now, in 1990 and at 205 pounds, I was ready to swim again. I was ready to whip myself back into shape.

More than one person at the time suggested that swimming wasn't always the best way to lose weight. The reasoning was that repeated exposure to the water caused your body to maintain a layer of blubber to keep you insulated from the cold. At first, this sort of made sense, but I couldn't help but picture real Olympic swimmers in my head. They certainly didn't look like whales to me. So I put those odd thoughts aside and enjoyed my pool time.

If I *were* retaining blubber, you would never have known it. Swimming several times a week and cutting down on the caloric intake had a decidedly positive effect. For about six weeks, life was good. Then, for the very first time as a card-carrying dieter, I met what was ultimately to become my arch nemesis:

ThanksGiving!!

This holiday just happens to be the basis of the Third Law of Dieting, "No diet, no matter how well it's going, can survive Thanksgiving." And not *just* Thanksgiving but also the entire forty-or-so day stretch from that gravy-laden Thursday to the hangover-clouded Monday after New Year's Day. Oh, it's a bad, bad time. This malevolent season has killed innumerable diets throughout the ages. Never before had I been concerned about this time of year (during that extraordinary part of my life, which I now refer to as *The Blissful Ignorance*).

My life would never be the same thereafter.

Before Thanksgiving, I'd actually managed to lose nearly twelve pounds, getting all the way down to 193.5. I felt pretty darn good with myself and didn't think a pumpkin pie or two (or six) could do *that* much damage. How wrong I was. I woke up from my feeding stupor on January 9, 1991 at 199.5.

A strange mixture of panic and relief set in at the sight of this particular number. Panic: that I'd essentially gone right back to two hundred. Relief: that the number at least still started with a *one*. Still, this situation was unacceptable. I vowed I would never again let myself go during the holidays like that. (Famous last words.)

As you know, nothing does a diet better than the turning of a new year. This (coupled with the firm resolve that carried over from the previous October) made 1991 a very good year. I continued to watch my eating, kept on swimming (even doing another mile!) and to my own utter astonishment, hit exactly 168 pounds on September 7. Take a look:

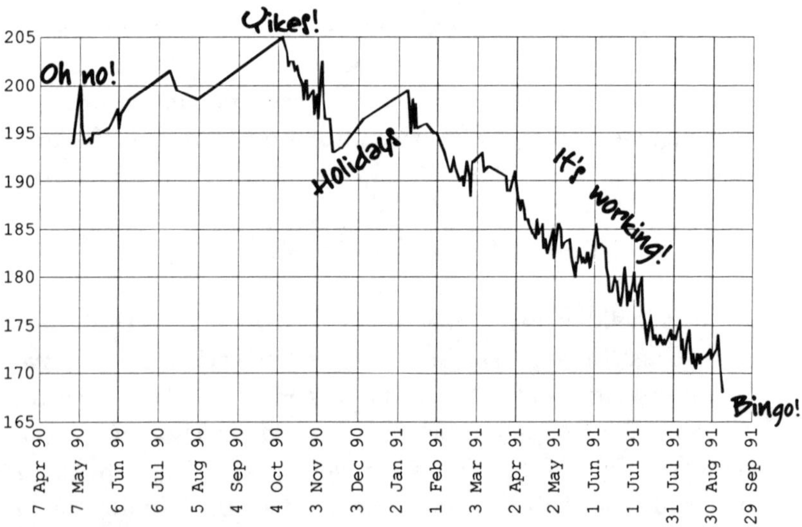

And he lived happily ever after.

If only! First of all, even more astonishing to me than losing thirty-seven pounds was the fact that I was still fat. True, true: I wasn't *as* fat. After all, I really did lose a lot of weight. But I still didn't look as good as I thought I should have. In spite of the compliments of friends, I still carried around a small spare tire and remained self-conscious about it. I certainly did not feel like I was to the point I could walk around in a bathing suit without feeling ill at ease. (Yes, ladies, men worry about this too. Oh sure, maybe not *all* men, but more than you think—and certainly more than most will let on about.)

Unfortunately, for me, the bathing suit problem became an issue much sooner than I ever thought it would. Even though the fall season was unmistakably upon us, about a month after hitting this all-time low weight, I got married. And about a month after *that*, I found myself in the Bahamas on our honeymoon. So at a time when my spare tire should have been comfortably hiding under thick November clothing, it suddenly found itself openly exposed to the Caribbean sun.

I *almost* got off scot-free. My wife Laura and I partook in a fair number of non-beach activities, all free of the risk of public exposure. We rented scooters to scoot about the island. We wandered into a casino and lost our free, hotel-provided ten-dollar chip at the roulette wheel. We even spent a wonderful seven or eight hours handcuffed in a small, dark room, learning about the benefits of time-share vacation properties.* In short, we were thoroughly enjoying ourselves all without the use of bathing suits. Unfortunately, that all came to an abrupt halt one day near the end of our trip when we signed ourselves up for a beach party.

Oh no. A beach party. This meant two things: 1) no shirt and 2) socializing with other humans. Being your basic born-and-bred geek, shirtless socializing just isn't my bag.

The party was on the other side of the island. A fair sized group had signed up for the trip. We piled into a bus and drove to the other side of the island. There were various beach activities, some group games, and (thankfully) plenty to drink. At one point during the party, we were instructed to split into groups: men and women. The women sat in chairs while the men stood a ways apart facing them. Music would be played and each guy in turn would strut his stuff for the cheering ladies in order to "win." (Whatever that meant.)

---

* Under no obligation whatsoever to buy anything, of course.

Oh no. Stuff-strutting. I had no stuff to strut. I never have and most certainly never will. But that was the least of my worries. What really hit home at that point was a single thought: how could I lose all that weight and still be flabby? Granted, on any given day I'd rather be 170 pounds-flabby than 205 pounds-flabby. But there on a Bahamian beach in an otherwise perfectly happy time, I just felt fat.

No one else cared, of course and in spite of it all, I had a really fun time, even if I didn't win.* It's just too bad all those pictures of stuff-strutting, shirtless Charlie somehow accidentally fell out of a locked suitcase and into the airplane toilet. Gosh, I have *no* idea how that happened.

A couple of weeks after we returned from the honeymoon, it was (unfortunately) Thanksgiving again. Wonderful. The holiday began, the expected forty-day feed-fest ensued, and when I woke up from this year's coma on January 1, 1992, I found I had climbed all the way back up to 189. *Sigh*. At first, I fought to keep the damage under 190:

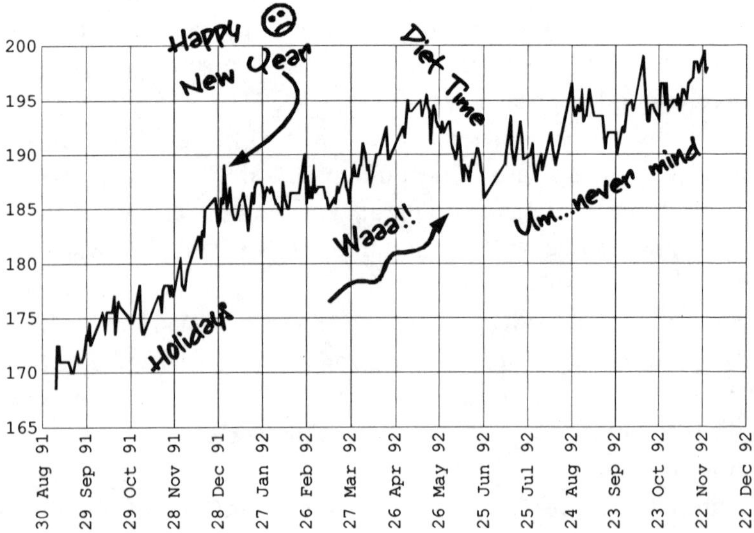

* Did I mention the alcohol?

When I realized this plan had zero chance of success, I switched gears and just tried to keep it below 200 for the year. And I actually managed it until—*wham!*—just like that, it was somehow Thanksgiving again. (Is it just me, or wasn't *last* Thanksgiving just one page ago? Time sure flies when you're eating too much.)

During this year's gauntlet, I continued to weigh myself almost daily, but threw out any pretense of dieting. After all, the holidays only come once a year: what else could I do? Nothing. So I ate and ate and ate. I simultaneously enjoyed and cursed every sugar plum and candy cane that passed my lips.

Therefore, it was with little surprise but no little shock that in mid-December the once unthinkable happened. I was back on the wrong side of the two hundred pound line. I had crossed the border and left Onederland behind.

This time the scale cheerfully reported 202.0. She took perverse pleasure in knowing that this—oh, yes—*this* was a Big One. This was the failure of nearly two years of hard work. Two years of eating better. Two years of exercising. Two years of sacrifice.

Hrmph! Two years of *nothing*. My diet had failed me, and my scale knew it.

"Scale, you must have this wrong," I pleaded. "This simply cannot be the right number! Please let me try again."

"Go right ahead!" she invited, barely able to keep a straight face.

She was, of course, eager to witness my dejected look again. (But not *too* eager. Scales do realize, after all, that their owners probably own heavy sledgehammers.) But my scale knows me better. She knows I won't do anything rash. I stepped back on.

Just as I feared: 202.0.

Sigh.

My diet had failed me.

Chapter 3

Why My Last Diet Failed Me

Let's say a neighbor of yours builds birdhouses as a hobby. You've watched him work out of his garage and have seen the fruits of his labor in his backyard. Happy birds flock from all around to nest. His aviary abodes are the envy of the neighborhood. One day you decide you'd like to give it a shot. You visit him, explain you're impressed by his handiwork, and ask if you can borrow his tools. "Of course," he cheerfully replies, as he lends you his hammers, saws, and various other craft-building implements. Thrilled by the prospect of constructing your own birdhouses, you march back to your own garage with great anticipation and excitement. Before long, you begin banging away on your very first project.

Um, make that your very *last* project. Your birdhouse looks like it was assembled by a blindfolded six-year-old using a butter knife. What happened? You used the exact same tools; shouldn't you get the exact same results?

We may only be on page fourteen but I'm about to let you in on the Really Big Secret. Ready for it? Well, ready or not, here goes: diets don't work.

That's right. I said diets don't work. I don't care if you're doing a traditional low-fat diet. I don't care if you're eating a case of grapefruit a week. It doesn't matter if you're on Atkins or South Beach or Weight Watchers or the latest craze. Diets simply do not work. [Author braces for attack.]

"How can you say that?"

"I know a guy who went low-carb and lost a hundred pounds!"

"A friend of mine ate Jenny Craig meals for six months and lost twenty pounds!"

"My mom lost thirty pounds on Weight Watchers!"

"Are you implying I didn't actually lose any weight?"

No, I'm not implying any of that. Whether you lost five, ten, fifty, or two hundred pounds: I believe you. You can trust me on that point. However, the operative word here is *you.* This is a very subtle yet enormously important distinction. And as the understanding of this distinction is the foundation for everything else in this book, let's make sure we're all on the same page before continuing. *You* lost five, ten, fifty, or two hundred pounds. Whether you accomplished this with a special diet or lots of exercise is completely and utterly beside the point. In no case did the diet somehow lose the weight for you. *You* lost the weight.

Let's turn back to our craft project for a moment. I hope it's obvious to you why our birdhouse didn't turn out as well as our neighbor's. Having possession of the tools is only half the equation. You obviously have to know what you're doing as well. In the same way, our diet isn't going to turn out as well as our neighbor's diet unless we have the right tools *and* we truly know what we're doing.

This is just how it works, folks. But for whatever reason we seem to be brainwashed into thinking the diet should do all the work. This even makes the birdhouse analogy worse, if you really think about it. A more accurate comparison would go something like this:

Thrilled by the prospect of building your own birdhouses, you march back to your own garage with great anticipation and excitement. You get the materials, lay out all the tools, and sit back. You wait and watch and nothing happens. You scratch your head, wondering when the birdhouse is going to show up. "These are the same tools that built my neighbor's birdhouses," you tell yourself, somewhat puzzled. After waiting a good long while for a birdhouse to appear spontaneously, you finally give up. "It's too hard. I tried everything but nothing worked."

The tools can't build birdhouses themselves. Yet that's exactly how most of us expect diets to work. We don't see them for what they truly are: tools. We prefer to see them as great magical train rides. We hand our tickets to the conductor, sit down, and we're whisked off to a wonderful, new place. All we have to do is read, or chat, or gaze out the window at the passing scenery. When we arrive at our destination, we hop off and we're there.

That's why your last diet failed you. It was never designed or intended to transport you to your destination. It was a tool: nothing more and nothing less. You were required to pick it up, wield it properly, and use it. The diet was no more responsible for your poor performance than your neighbor's tools were responsible for your pathetic birdhouse. If a diet ever "fails" you, it's for one of three reasons:

1. You never really picked it up at all.
2. You picked it up, but didn't use it right.
3. You used it right, but didn't finish using it.

The common factor being *you*.

Reason #3 is exactly what happened to me at the end of the last chapter. I certainly picked up the tool and I wielded it pretty well for the better part of a year. But, upon achieving my goal, I promptly dropped it. Is that the diet's fault? No. The diet was no more responsible for my failure than it was for my success. Yet I felt like the diet let me down because it should have somehow bestowed the power of tenacity upon me. Similarly, when I was successfully losing weight, the diet was getting all the credit. Odd how that works.

Consider the case of Chet.* He was your typical struggler and had tried many times to lose weight, with varying degrees of success. It's hard to tell why some things worked for him and others didn't. It's still harder to tell why, even when things *did* work, success never lasted. Then one time he struck upon a diet and found both great weight loss and long-lasting effects. Elated by his results, he could only assume that the diet was responsible. How could it not be? He'd tried and failed so many times before. *He* was a constant in the equation. The new diet was the variable.

What Chet didn't consider is what was going on inside him at the time. If you think about it, there's nothing "constant" about any of us. It may seem like we don't change from day to day, but we do. About every two to six weeks (depending on your age), your skin replaces itself. Look down at your body—what you now see before your eyes didn't even exist two months ago. Other body parts are hard at work too. Your stomach replaces its lining about every three days. Your liver replaces itself about once every two years. Believe it or not, even your skeleton replaces itself about once every ten years. And who knows how many brain cells you've killed so far by reading this book.

So even though Chet didn't feel like he changed at all, he really had. And perhaps he had changed just enough (both

---

* Names have been changed to protect the innocent.

mentally and physically—not that I personally make a great distinction between these two) that it was time for a diet to finally click. But to Chet's eyes, all he saw was magic. It never occurred to him that *he* made the diet work, and not the other way around.

Fast-forward a year or so. Chet has put back on about half the weight he lost. Like most of us do, he grew complacent and figured he could always lose it again, so what's the big deal? At this point, he decides to use his magic diet again, but for some reason, it's just not the same this time. Odd. It's the same diet. What's different now? Well, as you've probably already guessed, Chet is different. He's not the same person he was a year or so ago when he did it the first time. Suddenly the diet is the constant and the person is the variable. The diet doesn't (and didn't) work. Poor Chet.

We'll be exploring this and other related concepts a bit more later on. But before moving to the next page, I need to go on record by stating that the tool does indeed matter. For example, if for some reason I really *did* use a butter knife to cut wood, I should expect poor results no matter how skillfully the tool was used. Therefore, saying that *diets don't work* is not the same thing as saying *diets don't matter*. What you pick and how you pick it is a very important factor in the weight loss equation. That, too, we'll explore later. For now, let's look at our choice of tools.

Chapter 4

Pick a Diet, Any Diet

Okay, what do you want first, the good news or the bad news? Well, seeing as how I can't sit here and wait for you to respond, I'll just go ahead and choose for you. If you're thinking about going on a diet, the good news is you'll have no shortage of plans from which to choose. The bad news is you're guaranteed to pick the wrong one. (Of course, you won't find that out until *after* you've bought the stupid book for it.)

While I've done a lot of dieting in my day, I'm not the type of person who dejectedly (or triumphantly) proclaims, "I've tried everything." The reason is simple: I *haven't* tried everything. But I have tried more than a few and I've researched many others. I'd like to help you out by passing on what I've learned. (That way you can find out which diet is wrong for you by buying just this one stupid book.)

Since there's no possible way I can cover every diet program ever conceived, I won't even try. I'll attempt to discuss the most popular programs, but even that's a moving target. By the time this book is printed, the list is almost sure to be out of date. Lastly, be forewarned that I'm likely to say good things about the diet you hate and bad things about the diet you love. I am sorry. It's nothing personal. I'm just trying to make a fast buck here, that's all. ;^)

Before diving in, I'd like to begin with a few observations.

1. First and foremost, you're likely to find that diets are generally more alike than they are different. The greatest common factor is the simple fact that *all* of them force you to swim against the current. To put it another way, there's nothing natural about any of them. The human body fears famine and is therefore generally predisposed to eat as much as it can whenever it can. This is a wonderful trait to have when you don't know where your next meal is coming from. This is a terrible trait when your meals come thirty minutes apart.

2. I have yet to see a single diet that recommends eating lots of birthday cake and frosting. Very few of them recommend large volumes of cookies and ice cream. And I'll be damned if there's one that suggests eating one extra-large pepperoni pizza per day. (If you ever run across that one, *please* let me know about it at pizza@yourlastdiet.info.) It's pretty safe to say all diets avoid obviously bad foods in obviously large quantities.

3. They all tend to be more complex than they need to be. They go to great lengths to spell things out for you in the minutest detail. I can see only one explanation for this: no one would buy a diet's corresponding book if it were only three pages long. But think about it: if you have to memorize intricate plans and follow them to the letter, what are your real long-term chances of success?

You already know everything you need to know to lose weight. You need to eat right and exercise, plain and simple. Since this is far easier said than done, we often turn to popular diet programs for help. After all, if the diet worked for someone else, it just *has* to work for you too, right? And if it worked for them, your best bet is to run out and buy the book just to make sure you do it correctly.

But think about it: do you really need a book to tell you to eat more vegetables and fewer boxes of SnackWell's cookies? Do you really need a book to tell you that walking a mile a day is better for you than sitting in front of the TV for three hours? Do you really need someone to tell you to go for the salad instead of the super-sized fries?

I've heard the bizarre hypothesis that our nation's collective weight problem is due to a lack of basic nutritional understanding. Sorry, but I'm having more trouble swallowing that than a raw egg. If this were true, then fast food restaurants would have all gone out of business the day they began posting nutritional information. I can see it now. Chet walks into a McDonald's, stares at the posted Nutrition Chart for a few moments, then turns around and leaves in disgust. "Gosh, I didn't realize the Big Mac combo meal was chock full of fat and carbs! I think I'll head over to the Beansprout Hut for a tofu salad instead." Deep down inside we *know* what foods are bad and what amounts are wrong. The real trouble is we unconsciously choose to ignore the rules or (worse) consciously justify breaking them.

But I digress. Let's get back on track by summarizing my three observations: 1) diets are more alike than you might think; 2) no diets recommend clearly bad food in large volumes; and 3) you probably already know everything you need to know to lose weight, but read on anyway.

So without further ado, here is our diet program analysis, taking them in alphabetical order.

Dr Atkins' New Diet Revolution

The Atkins diet is the archetypal low carb diet. It wasn't the first, and it certainly won't be the last, but it definitely grabs the top spot in terms of mindshare.

The basic idea is that if you cut off the supply of your body's favorite food, you force it into using its vast reserves of stored fuel. Since your body's favorite food is sugar, you're forced to use a somewhat unconventional diet. Typically, this involves a pound of bacon for breakfast, a pound of bacon for lunch, and a pound of bacon for dinner. You're additionally allowed one dessert, such as one pound of Bacon Flavored Sugar Free Jell-O.

Just kidding. You can eat cheese too.

Seriously, though, the idea isn't quite as crazy as it sounds. After all, your body *is* storing all that fat for a reason: it's there for you to use when you really need it. The low carb diet simply generates that need. You're not meant to do it forever. You begin with a severely restricted level of carb intake to kick-start your body's fat burning engine. Once you begin losing weight, you gradually increase carb intake until your body finds its ideal level.

The most commonly cited downside to this diet is the lack of variety. The Atkins industry scoffs at this claim, pointing at the wide assortment of approved food items. For example, you can have peppered filet mignon with sautéed onions, or fire-grilled Maine lobster with white wine butter, or fresh wood-smoked venison sausage with a young Gouda cheese. Then, when you're flat broke after three days of this, you'll spend the rest of the diet eating dill pickles and Kraft Singles.

The upside is you really do get to eat many items forbidden on conventional diets. Whipping your own heavy cream and making sugar-free cheesecake is a real treat after years of fat-deprivation.

Verdict: Although it's not for everyone, there is sound science behind this approach. It may just work for you. Look past the hype and give it a try. I highly recommend it.

The Best Life

If you're a fan of *The Oprah Winfrey Show*, you don't need me to tell you about this one. And even if you haven't watched the show, you've probably heard about it already anyway: it's a best-seller. *The Best Life* program was developed by Bob Greene, a personal fitness and nutritional expert who's better known by his birth name, Oprah's Trainer.

Mr. Trainer has written several books and, along with his regular television appearances on the aforementioned show, has helped an untold number of people with their own weight issues.

This is his latest program. While admittedly I have not yet thoroughly researched it, I nonetheless feel I have a pretty good idea of what it entails. I've identified the five key steps:

1. Plop down on your living room couch.
2. Watch a Bob episode of *The Oprah Winfrey Show.*
3. Nod in agreement on his sound nutritional wisdom.
4. Laugh when Oprah makes a joke about weight or food.
5. Remain inspired for up to an hour after the show.

After the inspiration wears off, head to the kitchen, whip up some Hamburger Helper for dinner, and resume your normal not-so-best life.

Verdict: In all seriousness, his program is based on solid nutrition, involves good amounts of exercise, and getting your head on straight. I highly recommend it.

Body for Life

This is a program designed by Bill Philips. It's fundamentally another eat-right-and-exercise program, with the emphasis on purchasing items from his extensive line of nutritional products. Um, I mean, with the emphasis on exercise! And by exercise, I do mean *exercise.*

Here's the program in a nutshell: your diet is broken down into three main parts: 40% carbs, 40% protein, 20% fat.

Your exercise is broken down into two types: bodybuilding and aerobic. The diet keeps you both balanced and fueled. The bodybuilding is for shaping and the aerobic exercise is for weight loss. You stay on the program six days a week. You get one day off to do whatever you want.

The hallmark of the Body for Life program is the before-and-after combo picture. The book (and web site) is filled with photographs of extraordinarily successful participants. The typical "before" picture for a guy shows a bearded, flabby, Michelin Man who has a look on his face as if he just found out his puppy died. Afterwards, he is a smiling, well lit, oiled-up, Mr. Olympian, daring you to take the challenge yourself next year. The typical "before" picture for a woman is similar. She is pear-shaped, has her hair pulled up, and legs that touch each other far more than they should. Afterwards, she looks like her real body was snatched by aliens and replaced with a supermodel. The pictures really are quite amazing to look at, not to mention inspirational. When you see someone go from Pillsbury Doughboy to Bodybuilding Champion in just twelve weeks, you can't help but get motivated.

Does it work? Of course it does! How could focused eating patterns and working out six days a week *not* work? Will it work for you? Of course it won't! Because you're a regular person, and regular people don't make those kinds of body changes in just twelve weeks. The basic workout alone will not fetch the kinds of results shown in the after photos. So don't go into this type of program thinking that by drinking enough Myoplex shakes, you'll just wake up buff one morning. It will take lots of work, but the results have to be worth it.

Verdict. I highly recommend you get off the couch, buy a bench and a good set of free weights, and give this one a try. Take the challenge!

Detox Diet

Unlike many of the other diets here, this one doesn't have a corporate sponsor. It's an approach, not a product. The basic idea is that our modern diet is filled with crap and every once in a while you need to clean your filters. Detox diets are also known as cleansing diets.

In general, "crap" is defined as "everything you love." So you can say goodbye to cheeseburgers, ice cream, pepperoni pizza, cookies, soda pop, onion rings, pancakes, corndogs, and—I can barely utter the words—French fries. What you're left with is a diet rich in cardboard and Styrofoam.

The good news is you don't do this forever. Generally, a week or two just once or twice a year is all that's necessary to keep your parts running smoothly. Proponents say it's essential to keeping your body free of the toxins so prevalent in the modern food supply: additives, preservatives, artificial this, synthetic that. Critics say the body is already well suited for getting rid of this stuff all by itself. Still, it is just a temporary thing, and if giving up cheese, bologna, and Ding Dongs for a week is bad, then I don't know what's good.

Verdict. Go ahead and bite the bullet. Swap McDonald's for broccoli one week and see if you don't feel better. I highly recommend it.

The Food Guide Pyramid

Most of us grew up with the four food groups. The concept? The healthiest diet consisted of equal portions of dairy, meats, breads, and jellybeans. Hmmm...maybe it wasn't jellybeans. I honestly can't remember anymore. That's because it was replaced years ago with the Food Guide Pyramid.

Instead of a nice square, with four equal parts, the pyramid dictates more realistic proportions. At the bottom of the pyramid you find the grains. If I recall correctly, you're supposed to have forty-seven servings a day of foods in this group. The next two groups sit side by side, just above the base. On one side is the vegetable group. On the other side is the fruit group. [What's that? No, sir, I don't believe Twinkies are technically a fruit. Please hold all questions until the end of the tour.] The next level up contains the dairy and meat groups. And then, at the very top, is apparently the salt and pepper group. At least that's what the picture looks like. In fact, there's salt and pepper sprinkled all over this thing. That doesn't make any sense. Oh wait, that's not salt and pepper. It's fat and sugar. My bad.

To me, the pyramid is the quintessential example of why the simple "eat right and exercise" directive doesn't work for most people. The two main problems of the pyramid are: 1) it makes sense; and 2) it's not sexy. It's like a financial planner. You know it's sensible, and that if you follow the advice, you'll be far better off in the long run. But most people simply aren't that self-motivated. It's far easier to grab another bag of chips than to turn your life around after reading about the pyramid on a bread wrapper.

From what I've gathered, nutrition professionals almost seem dismayed that, on the whole, we didn't get any slimmer after the pyramid was released. I can't imagine what they expected would happen. This just doesn't seem to me like the kind of thing that falls into the "if you build it, they will come" category. Most of it falls into the "you already know this" category. The pyramid's official web site offers helpful information, like how there's more added sugar in a frosted slice of cake than in a slice of bread. (Really?) Or this: "Grape and orange sodas don't count as fruit juice."

Sigh.

I don't know. Maybe this stuff isn't as obvious to some people as it is to me. After all, this is the same society that prints "Warning: may cause drowsiness" on sleep-aids. All cynicism aside, the pyramid approach is quite sound. *If* you've made up your mind you're ready to do something *and* you're looking for a sound, no-frills program, then following the pyramid will definitely get you results.

Verdict: I *would* like to recommend this, but unfortunately, the traditional Food Guide Pyramid was discontinued in 2005. If the government can't recommend it, neither can I. Luckily, they replaced it with MyPyramid. Sure, it may still look like your basic Egyptian tomb, but it makes a lot less sense to me. The old one was wide at the base (eat those foods most) and narrow at the top (eat those the least). How simple. The new pyramid takes a different approach. Now you get colored vertical bands depicting the proportions of each food group. The colors intuitively represent each group. In order, from left to right:

- Orange: The sandwich group.
- Green: The lasagna group.
- Red: The side order group.
- Yellow: The breakfast cereal group.
- Blue: The seafood group.
- Purple: The candy and donut group.

The final difference between the old and new pyramids is the depiction of a human figure climbing up stairs on the left side of the new pyramid. This visual clue reminds you to eat on the upper floor of the restaurant, if one is available.

Hoodia Gardonii

This is it, folks. This is the true miracle you've been waiting for. It's all natural. It comes from a faraway land. It's everything you've ever wanted in a weight loss product.

Here's how it works. Simply slash your caloric intake by fifty percent and exercise at least eight hours per week. If you do that—and keep a bottle of this stuff on the counter—the weight will melt right off. Now I'm sure you're asking yourself, "Where can I get some of this miracle-in-a-bottle?" Don't worry. It's easy!

1. Set up a new e-mail account.
2. Wait twelve hours.
3. Make a purchase from one of the thousands of reputable vendors who've contacted you solely in the interest of your long-term health.

Verdict: Hey, ten thousand snake oil salesmen can't be wrong. If you're ready to lose some weight (and susceptible to placebos) then I highly recommend this one.

Intolerance Diets

In the third movie* of the popular series, *Harry Potter and the Prisoner of Azkaban*, Professor Snape asks the class if they know the difference between a werewolf and an animagus. Hermione responds that an animagus can turn into an animal at will and a werewolf has no choice.

Welcome to the life of the Intolerance Dieter, the werewolf of the weight loss world. While most of us choose to diet of our own free will, people with food intolerances or allergies have no choice. A normal person can cheat a bit on their diet and make it up the next day. The food intolerant or allergic person can cheat a bit and die. Talk about motivation.

I have to admit there are times when I wish I had that kind of motivation. Imagine how easy it would be to resist temptation if you knew the consequences of caving in were two days of intense illness. Intolerance dieters *do not cheat.* Of course, this is about the same thing as wishing I could get in a crippling accident just so I could park in the handicapped spot. I don't *really* want a food intolerance. I'm one of the lucky few *not* allergic to anything whatsoever. (But my hair is falling out at an alarming rate, so I wouldn't completely consider myself leading a charmed life.)

Verdict. If you have no food intolerances, don't go out and get one. I do not recommend this.

Jenny Craig

If you want to go on a diet but don't know your way around your own kitchen, this one just might be the ticket. The basic eating plan is nothing new at all. It's everything you've read about focusing on grains, vegetables, fruits, and other "good"

---

* Oh, man! Have you heard what happens in the sixth book yet?

foods. You avoid high fat foods and eat in moderation. If you can't do that on your own, and have a healthy disposable income, then Jenny Craig just might be for you.

The meals are a small part of it. What Jenny Craig really offers most is help. If you're like most people, you probably *can't* do it on your own. Using Jenny Craig Centers or Jenny Direct (an at-home program with personalized phone calls), their consultants just might be that extra boost you've been looking for.

You typically spend your first six months eating the pre-packaged meals. The going rate seems to be around $80 per week. It's left as an exercise to the reader to calculate if this is out of line or not. The three oft-cited drawbacks are:

1. The pre-packaged meal approach doesn't work well when you're on the road or entertaining guests.
2. It's easy to grow dependent on them and not properly learn how to fend for yourself in the wild.
3. You run the constant danger of having to appear on Oprah in a two-piece.

If you can get past these issues, you just may have found what you've been looking for.

Verdict. If having your own food consultant is what you think you need, and you don't have time to prepare your own meals, you may be quite happy with Jenny Craig. I highly recommend it.

Orlistat

If you don't recognize this, you might know it by its over-the-counter name *Alli*. It was an instant hit by dieters desperate for another Magic Pill.

The basic idea of Orlistat is to block the body's absorption of dietary fat. Under normal gastrointestinal operations, triglycerides are broken down into absorbable fatty acids. This operation is completed with the help of an enzyme called *pancreatic lipase.* Orlistat blocks this enzyme so the fats you eat just pass on through. If your body doesn't *absorb* the fat then it won't *get* fat.

I hope you see the problem with this. Sticking to a new diet is hard enough when you have to do all the work yourself. Imagine what you would do with a crutch like this. You'll think, "Oh, I can keep eating all the fat I want! It won't stick!" Are you prepared to take this for the rest of your life? Does anyone know what the long-term effects of blocking pancreatic lipase are? Do you really think you'll keep the weight off after you stop taking this?

Most importantly Orlistat is not without side effects (or "treatment effects" as they call them.) If you've heard of this product then you've certainly already heard about the side effects. I know this is mostly a humor book, but I'll refrain from capitalizing on the topic. Come on—that'd be like shooting fish in a barrel.

However, if for some reason you haven't heard about the side effects, I'll try to explain. Hmmm ... Let me think for a second. Okay, I've got one. Let's say you're at work and you go to a meeting where everyone has brought along his or her bagpipes. The meeting is rolling along fine until suddenly, and without warning, your bagpipes start playing *Kelly the Boy from Killane* all by themselves. If this kind of scenario strikes fear into your heart, then you might want to avoid this product.

Verdict: If you're willing to live on the edge a bit and are at the end of your dieting rope, I suppose you might find help here. If that's your situation, then I recommend trying this.

The Peanut Butter Diet

You know, I really like peanut butter...I mean, I know that's not profound or nothin'...Heck! We ALL do. But for me, I think it goes much more beyond that.*

---

* My apologies to Gary Larson.

When I first heard of the peanut butter diet, I was quite ecstatic. Just imagine! Being able to lose weight eating one of the bestest foods ever created.

I'm serious about that too. I can't even imagine a world without peanut butter. I like all types too. From the raw paste you get from grinding your own in the store to the smoothest, lard-laden, trans-fat enriched commercial stuff, solely meant to be spread on Wonder bread with grape jelly. It's all good—and it's always been one of my bigger weaknesses. It's not unusual to find a big jar of it on my desk at work. In fact, "on my desk" is where it spends the least amount of time as I typically keep the jar strapped on my muzzle like a feedbag, much to the alarm of my co-workers.

So you can see how a peanut butter diet seemed too good to be true. As it turned out, it *was* too good to be true. The basic idea of the Peanut Butter diet is to eat less and exercise. (I don't know where people find such crazy ideas.) As you might expect from the name, it *does* involve peanut butter. But my disappointment came when I learned the diet only called for four to six tablespoons of peanut butter a day, just to ward off hunger. I could have sworn it said forty-six tablespoons a day, which would have been more my speed. Case in point: I actually ate an entire food service sized can of the stuff in two weeks—all by myself. And I wonder why I have a weight problem.

But back to the diet at hand. The basic idea is you eat in moderation, exercise a fair amount, throw in a little peanut butter to ward off hunger, and there you go. The total caloric intake is exactly what you'd expect from any reasonable diet.

Verdict: Like so many other plans, this diet does help you control portions and encourages exercise. I highly recommend it over diets that forbid The Butter.

Dr. Phil's Ultimate Weight Solution

As you might expect from a psychologist, this program starts in your head. His approach is all about changing yourself from the "inside out." In short, if you can fix your head, your body will follow. Of course, that's the real trick isn't it?

The research for the book is based on the years he spent counseling overweight patients. That alone has to be good stuff. My only worry is transference. Namely, is reading a book just as good as seeing an actual therapist on a regular basis? I believe it would be far easier to get real results in a private doctor/patient environment. You just can't get that level of service from a book. I could be wrong. I often am.

On the positive side, he does try to help you get control of your emotions and triggers. He does recommend you get all of the junk out of your pantry. And he rightly states that without exercise, there isn't much hope for any of us. I can't say anything bad about that.

Verdict: While a book is no substitute for a one-on-one relationship with a professional therapist, there are some sound ideas here. I highly recommend it.

The Pizza Diet

There is no pizza diet, remember? E-mail me if you find it—especially if it involves very thin crusts and lots of pepperoni. And if the pepperoni's on top and crispy, then all the better.

Verdict: I can't help but highly recommending make-believe diets. It's what separates us from the animals.

The Pritikin Principle

With dozens of new diets coming on the scene practically every month, it's easy for older diets to get buried in the pile. The Pritikin diet encourages the participant to, "Take it easy, don't over-exert yourself, and keep eating the 40% fat American diet of eggs, beef, and the like, until you die."

Oh, wait. Never mind. That's what they *don't* want you to do. Nathan Pritikin came up with this plan in the 1950s when he was diagnosed with heart disease and wanted to find a path back to health through better eating. He ended up crafting a program based on caloric density. Foods high in fat contain more calories by volume than low-fat counterparts. As an illustration, picture one pound of peanuts vs. one pound of popcorn. The peanuts will clock in at around 2,600 calories. The same amount of popcorn comes in at about 3,000 calories. But look at the difference in volume: 3.2 cups of peanuts vs. 100 cups of popcorn. You *may* fit three cups of peanuts down your gullet but there's no chance you'll cram one hundred cups of popcorn down there. That's the basic idea: fill up on foods that won't weigh you down.

This means eating lots of vegetables, fruits, and unrefined carbohydrates. It means small amounts of animal protein. Fish is preferred over poultry and poultry over red meat. In fact, they recommend red meat no more than once a month if you can help it. Once a month? Sheesh! I'm having trouble limiting red meat to no more than once every three hours. Personally, I think I have a way to go before I'm ready for something like this.

Verdict: A diet like this may require some drastic changes. But, as the saying goes, drastic times call for drastic measures. As with the Detox diet, there's nothing wrong with adding more veggies to your plate. I highly recommend it.

The Scarsdale Diet

This is another low carb diet, but unlike Atkins, which emphasizes tailoring the program to each individual, the Scarsdale diet enforces a plan to be followed to the letter. In addition to being low carb, it's also low calorie. How low? Well, how does 700 calories per day sound to you? That's right, 700. Hell, my left leg requires 700 calories a day. I don't know what the rest of my body would do. If the extremely low calorie plan wasn't enough, it also requires beginning the day with grapefruit. That was enough for me. I don't like grapefruit at all. (But I do like Fresca. Does that count?)

Verdict: If you're *really* ready for results and can handle a militant program, this just might be for you. Plenty of people out there swear by this one. I highly recommend it.

Slim Fast

This plan employs the revolutionary weight loss approach of eating fewer calories and exercising. (I'm still amazed at how there are so many different ways of losing weight.) The basic idea is that if you replace your large, delicious meals with eight ounces of flavored milk, you're going to lose weight. The third meal, dinner, should be sensible.

I don't think anyone's ever put this into perspective better than Rosie O'Donnell. She once mocked in a stand-up routine, "A shake for breakfast, a shake for lunch, and then a sensible meal for dinner. A *sensible* meal! If I could eat a sensible meal, I wouldn't need the @#$!ing Slim Fast to begin with."

She has a point, you know.

Does Slim Fast work? Sure it does. It forces you to reduce your caloric intake, and as we all know, that makes you lose weight. But then again which diet doesn't make you do that? There's nothing remarkably special or magical about it or the products.

I recall one day standing in the kitchen at work where a co-worker had a six-pack of the ready-made shakes. While we were chatting, I glanced at a can to see what it was made out of (primarily skim milk, water, and chocolate). Two thoughts popped in my head: how much did you pay for this, and why not just make your own chocolate milk at home? Drop a Flintstone's vitamin in it, and you're all set. If it's all about replacing a meal with a lower-calorie drink, what more do you need?

That said, they do offer a rather wide range of products, and the focus is still on eating less. And as we all know, that will always help you lose weight,

Verdict: If you like the program, the foods, and the prices, Slim Fast can get you results. I highly recommend it.

The South Beach Diet

The South Beach diet is, at heart, a low carb plan. Given that, the diet is quick to distance itself from the negative connotations associated with Atkins and other "crazy" fad diets.

They've actually been quite successful at that, to be honest. Ask the average Joe on the street what South Beach is, you'll rarely get "low carb" as an answer.

Where the programs differ is in their core principles. South Beach recommends you avoid refined carbs. The Atkins diet, on the other hand, recommends you avoid refined carbs. South Beach severely restricts the intake of these foods during the first phase of the diet. Atkins goes the other way and instead severely restricts intake of these foods during the first phase of the diet. South Beach allows fruits and whole grains later in the diet. Atkins, in contrast, allows fruits and whole grains later in the diet.

No, you're not seeing double. I'm going out of my way to make a point: they actually *do* have a lot of the core principles in common, and that's not a bad thing. In my mind, it lends more weight to both of them. They both distinguish good carbs from bad carbs. The real difference is South Beach makes this a gigantic marketing point, Atkins doesn't.

South Beach does recommend you avoid saturated fats while Atkins doesn't separate saturated and unsaturated fats. (Although both tell you to avoid trans-fats—long before it was fashionable to do so.) They also count carbs differently. South Beach counts portions while Atkins counts grams. Lastly, South Beach generally gets you through the phases more quickly. It's a longer process with Atkins.

Verdict: Bombarding our systems with foods that cause non-stop sugar highs is bad. South Beach helps you fix that problem. I highly recommend it.

Weight Watchers

This program has been around for over forty years. If you've never heard of it then you really need to get out more. Weight Watchers is not about restricting specific foods, but instead emphasizes eating in moderation. This is done through a simplified calorie-counting mechanism called POINTS. Calories alone can be hard to count, especially when you're counting hundreds or thousands of them. Also, calories do not take into account what *types* of food you're eating. Pure calorie counting won't distinguish 100 calories of carrots from 100 calories of carrot cake. The POINTS system generates a small, easy to use number by taking calories, fat, and fiber all into account.

Fans of Weight Watchers swear it's the easiest way to keep track of what they're eating. It does require you to track every M&M that passes your lips without dictating, "You can never, ever eat M&Ms again." As long as everything balances at the end of the day, you're good. Critics find the counting tedious and hard to continue for long periods. Heck, even its *proponents* can tire of counting points day after day, week after week, month after month.

Weight Watchers itself has recognized this and devised an alternate "no counting" plan. If you tried Weight Watchers in the past, liked the general idea, but didn't like the POINTS system, you might want to give it another look.

Another hallmark of Weight Watchers is the group meeting. The idea is that if you gather once a week with dieters just like you, you may find the support you need that you'd never find on your own. From what I've heard, they take great pains to emphasize, "It's not about the weight." This seems odd to me given the company name begins with "Weight" and they make you weigh in every week. I don't know about you, but that sounds to me like weight has a lot to do with it.

Does it work? Weight Watchers has a huge fan base and most will tell you it's the only plan that's ever worked for them. In fact, it works every single time they try it—first, second, eighth, ninth, etc. That is to say, just like *all* plans, it works *if you stick to it.* And as we've already explored, "sticking to it" isn't something the diet can bestow upon you.

Verdict: Weight Watchers has been around a long time and helped many people, even if it is the same people getting the same help repeatedly. Go to their web site and read a few of the success stories. You may find inspiration. I highly recommend it.

The Zone

The Zone was created by Dr. Barry Sears. In spite of his recommendation that forty percent of calories come from carbohydrates, his plan has many similarities to low carbohydrate diets. Foremost in my mind is the shared idea of getting the right blood sugar levels. Just like Atkins, Sears found it somewhat odd that the country became collectively more obese exactly during the time when low-fat diets ruled. The reason is due to the fact that *low fat* typically implies *high carb*, and the body turns carbs into basic sugars more quickly than any other food type. And if feeding your body its favorite fuel wasn't enough, you actually *emphasize* these food types. Your body doesn't know what to do with all the excess energy and has no choice but to save it for later, in the form of your well-padded posterior.

Another similarity is the idea that fats in a meal (specifically monounsaturated fats, such as olive oil) can help you feel full and therefore function as a natural appetite suppressant. This means less work on the pancreas and eventually your stored fat gets converted back into fuel.

As with all diets, proponents swear by it. Critics find it unnatural or even unhealthy, typically citing too much protein and not enough long-term study on the effects.

Verdict: Don't get over-worried about "long-term" effects. I doubt you're planning on doing the diet for twenty years straight, anyway. Keeping blood sugars in line is a good thing. I highly recommend it.

In Conclusion. . .

It was simultaneously fascinating, disturbing, and mind-blowing doing the research for this chapter. I mean, I knew there were a lot of diets out there. Heck, we all know that. But until you *really* start digging into it, the full impact doesn't really hit you. Go to Amazon.com and do a search on the word "diet." I did just that one afternoon and fetched 176,134 results. If you could somehow read one book every single day, you would be reading books for the next five hundred years. It's no wonder Susan Powter begged us to stop the insanity.

The astute reader may have noticed I highly recommended every single program listed. Shouldn't I just pick the best one and recommend that one to you? Well, no, I shouldn't and there's an astoundingly good answer why: *I don't know you*. I have no idea who you are, what you're like, or how you've lived. I don't know your medical history, your family history, or even your financial history. I don't know what foods you enjoy, despise, or are deathly allergic to. How on earth can I recommend the best diet for you?

It doesn't take a huge leap of logic to grasp, how does *anyone* know the best diet to recommend for you? The happy, smiling people on the late-night infomercials don't know *you*. Bob Greene doesn't know *you*. The authors of these 176,134 books don't know *you*. Yet it's interesting how they all seem to know exactly what will work for *you*. Go figure.

Of course, we all share the physiological basics. It's not statistically wrong to take the results of a given sample size and extrapolate the results to a larger population. That is to say, if the majority of participants on a given program lost a given amount of weight in a given amount of time then there's a chance you will too. But what we tend to ignore is the fact that the majority of people actually *fail*. They try and fail (or they try, succeed and *then* fail). But one way or another, the majority succumbs to instinct and situation—the instinct that drives us to eat: the situation where we have all the food we'll never need, and then some. Think about it. What else would explain why every single program comes with the exact same qualifier?

"Anne lost 45 lbs in six weeks." (*Results not typical.*)
"Barb lost nine inches in 14 days." (*Results not typical.*)
"Carmen lost four dress sizes!" (*Results not typical.*)

We never stop to consider the underlying meaning of this phrase. It's really just another way to say, "No results *quite* typical." We don't want the truth. We can't handle the truth. We just want someone to hand us the answer so we don't have to think about it.

And that's exactly why we've never (and will never) run out of so-called "solutions" to our collective problem. This may or may not be bad news to you. Because if you've tried the all the diets discussed in this chapter and still haven't found something that works for you, take heart. You can still choose The 3 Hour Diet, the Abs Diet, the Beverly Hills diet, or even Cabbage Soup. There's also Carbohydrates Addicts, Dr. Gott, Eat Right for Your Type, The Fat Smash Diet, The Fiber35 Diet, and Food Combining & Digestion. No? Still haven't found the one you want? Don't worry! There's also the G.I. Diet, Grapefruit Diets, the Hay Diet, Juice Fasts, or Liquid Diets. You can go Low Fat, Low Sodium, Macrobiotic, Mediterranean, Neanderthin, Negative Calories, or take the Perricone Prescription. And if none of these trips your trigger, there's always Protein Power, Richard Simmons, Sugar Busters, or the Secrets of the Stars. Shall I go on?

It truly is insane. How many more books do we need? How many more plans? How much more advice? We already have upwards of fifty *million* pages on the subject in print and yet two thirds of the United States is still overweight. Clearly, something isn't working here, folks.

For now, all I want you to take away from this chapter is this: no diet is a sure thing. The only sure thing is *you*. Decide for yourself which tool is the best fit but never expect the tool itself to do the work. That's exactly what most everyone else has already done (and you saw where it got them).

Chapter 5

It Just Doesn't Get Any Better Than This

After my fright of returning to the two hundreds in December of 1992, I decided to kick off the New Year by starting another diet program. How original. I was determined to find a way to get back to where I was just two short years before.

And just what exactly *is* it about a new year? Why are our lives filled suddenly with renewed hope and promise just at the mere tick of the clock? Have you ever joined a health club in January? First, you wait in line to join. Then you wait in line to change clothes. After that, you wait in line for an unoccupied stair machine or for a lane to open in the pool. You wait for all the other Resolutioneers who are there for the exact same reason you are: that magical, mystical tick of the clock that brought the previous year to a close.

I may not know how it is we're able to wipe the slates clean so easily, but I'm not going to complain about it either. I quite enjoy the feeling myself. I'm sure a big part of it (for me at any rate) is finally getting through the holidays and restoring some sense of order in my life. Andy Williams had a good song, but "It's the Most *Disruptive* Time of the Year" would have painted a more accurate picture. The New Year heralds a "return to normalcy." (Normal, that is, as long as you don't count our impractical New Year Resolutions.)

January 1993 was no different for me. I climbed back on the wagon and by March had lost about ten pounds—hitting a low of 192.5 on April 16. Unfortunately, it wasn't going to get any better than this. Not for a long, *long* time. I bounced around this "low" point for a couple months, desperately trying to get back on track, but it wasn't to be. In June, I hit two hundred again and by July, it was all but over.

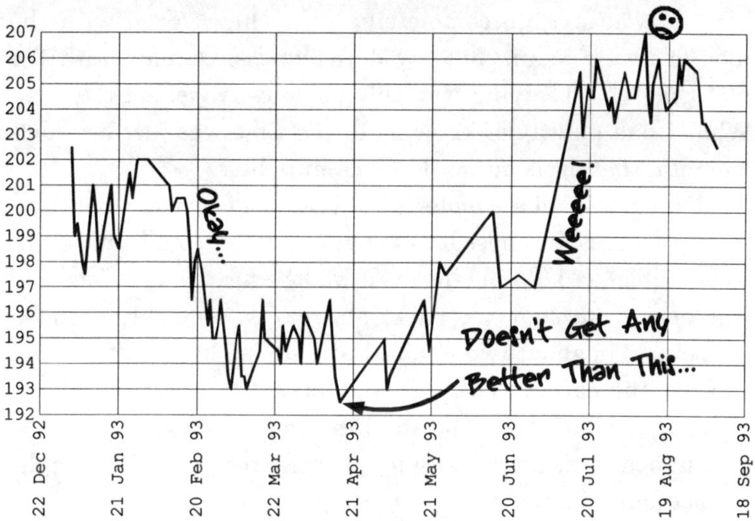

I may have been down, but I wasn't yet out. Undaunted, on September 7, I declared yet another Day One. I weighed in that day at 202.5 pounds, which ironically was my starting weight back in January. But this time (and for the first time), I took a bunch of body measurements. The key measurement for me is what many euphemistically call "waist" but what we all know really means "big fat gut." It was 42½ inches. I don't recall ever measuring it before, but this seemed like a big enough number for me. It was time to get serious again. I did just that and things went well enough for a short while but somehow by November 22 (just before you-know-when) I was right back up to 203. Argh!

Now I'd seen numbers like this before. (In fact, I'd gone all the way up to 207 the previous August.) But something about this number hit hard. It was, of course, another failure. But I think that for the first time ever I now realized *failure was the norm.* Suddenly I was aware that *I had better get used to this.* Losing weight and keeping it off isn't as easy as it sounds. There must be other forces at work.

Seeing a big, bad number on the scale causes one of two distinct reactions. Either you screw yourself up for another go at it or you give up completely. I may have toyed with the idea of trying again, but my dejectedness, coupled with the fact that Thanksgiving was only days away, sealed the deal. What I had no way of knowing at the time was just how detrimental that decision would turn out to be.

I'm sure I had a wonderful Christmas, because when I returned to consciousness on January 3, 1994, I had hit an all-time high of 210.5. Pushing over into the next weight "decade" was enough to snap me back into reality. I quickly dropped six pounds in about two weeks, but I gained back half of them shortly thereafter. Then on January 24 wrote down my weight for what would be the last time in six months. This was unheard of, after so many years of recording my weight almost daily. I must have really stopped caring.

In August of 1994, I embarked on (what turned out to be) a series of "dietlets." The dietlet is wonderful: you start it on Monday; you end it on Friday. The next week you do it all over again. It's marked by a drastic drop in daily caloric intake on Monday and pigging out on Friday night. It's a great way to gain weight slowly and draws a perfect saw tooth graph. Of course, no one typically *plans* on going on a dietlet. You swear each Monday—each new "Day One"—that this one is going to be *the one.* But you're at a point in your life, both physically and psychologically, where you're not ready for it to click. You haven't flipped the switch in your head yet, so you haven't truly resolved to do anything about the problem. It may certainly be that your higher brain functions are shouting, "Hey Stupid! Don't you think losing some weight would be a good idea about now?" But the rest of your system simply isn't cooperating. The only response it sends back is, "Send down more tortilla chips."

For me, my system *definitely* wasn't cooperating. As I scan through my notes taken from this period, I see myself constantly bemoaning how things are not progressing according to plan. This culminated in January 1995 when I hit 219.5 and merely wrote, "This was extremely frightening to see." I'd never seen a number that size staring up at me from between my two big toes. (In fact, I barely even saw it then, what with having to lean out waaaay over my gut just to see the scale.)

Two hundred and nineteen point five! I suddenly found myself pining for the days when I thought 205 was a big number. How much worse could this get? And why was I so unable to do anything about it? I'm a reasonably intelligent person. I understand the mechanics of caloric theory. But why did I have seemingly no control over it?

This perceived lack of control is what someone looking in from the outside would have great difficulty understanding. It's easy to play armchair quarterback, shouting out various plays. "Don't eat so much!" "Exercise some more!" "Show a little willpower!"

Willpower! That's a good one. Anyone who has ever found oneself in one of these private feeding frenzies will immediately know that willpower has nothing to do with it. This is no more a failure of will than getting knocked out by a falling rock is a failure of strength. But we don't look at it that way. All we see is someone standing in the kitchen late at night with a ravenous look in the eyes. Our test subject is standing over a bag of Doritos, or a box of cookies, or a tub of ice cream. Our test subject is mindlessly shoveling food into his or her mouth. Our test subject probably isn't even hungry. In fact, it's a safe bet this person isn't even happy. And when it's over, regret will set in—bad.

The human body, like the rest of the known universe, is comprised of atoms. In fact, ninety-nine percent of your body is made up of just four elements: hydrogen, oxygen, carbon, and nitrogen. The remaining one percent is comprised of some thirty odd other elements, including some you'd expect (like calcium) along with things you'd never dream of (would you believe gold, arsenic, and uranium?). Unbeknownst to you, the seven billion billion billion atoms that make up your body have decided they want to assimilate the atoms in that tub of ice cream. These atoms have unanimously elected not to consult you. They will get their ice cream. Resistance is futile.

Oh, you can try and fight it for a while, but it does more harm than good. No, you have to be nice to your atoms or they'll get mad and go be somebody else instead.

So you can see how our test subject has been reduced to nothing more than a biomechanical machine—signals in the body overriding all senses, subverting all conscious control. This is why I believe overeating is not always your fault. At least not the way we usually think of "fault."

Of course, if this were a legal case, it would *definitely* be your fault. No one forced you to do it. You were wide-awake during the entire episode. What judge or jury would take more than two seconds to declare your guilt? Your only hope would lie in a skilled courtroom attorney who might be able to have you declared "not guilty by reason of insanity." If a videotape of your feeding frenzy had been admitted as evidence, it just might be possible to prove—or at the very least, demonstrate—that you were somehow completely bonkers at the time of the crime.

"Look at him, your honor. He's an automaton. Even though he *knows* he shouldn't be doing this and will *hate* himself in the morning, he continues his behavior. He's as mindless as a shark, devouring anything that comes within six inches of his gaping maw. He is clearly out of his mind and I recommend psychological help immediately. But first, I move we recess for lunch."

If you really think about it, this has all the earmarks of an addiction. What person with an alcohol addiction thinks, "Gee, you know what I'd like to do today? Get drunk again! Oh how I enjoy it so!" What person with a drug addiction gains immense satisfaction out of their problem? What person of sound mind actually *wants* to continue this kind of self-destructive behavior—and to do so repeatedly—even when faced with mountains of negative reinforcement?

Yet we, as society, do not view it as such. If a person, for whatever reason, becomes an alcoholic, then we say he or she has an identifiable disease. Alcohol, as everyone knows, is a mind-altering substance. And mind-altering substances are where *real* problems lie. Not something like eating a few cookies. Cookies are good and tasty treats—not addictive substances. Besides, who has ever heard of someone driving his or her car through the garage door because of a cookie overdose? Who has lost their job over their cookie problem? Who has ever accidentally gotten pregnant after a plate of Christmas cookies? Who ever woke up in jail after an all-night cookie bender?

You see, the issue lies in what we think of as an addictive substance. We prefer to view things in black or white, because doing so makes life easier to deal with. But life isn't simple. I don't believe a substance is either *addictive* or *not addictive*. I simply cannot believe that a machine with trillions of moving parts will behave in such simplistic terms. I prefer to think addictive chemicals fall along a continuum.

I mean, look at the molecular formula of alcohol (C_2H_5OH) compared to that of glucose ($C_6H_{12}O_6$). Is it *so* inconceivable that they might *both* have the potential to be addictive—but only to different degrees? Your body consumes chemicals, processes chemicals, and reacts to chemicals. Some are mildly addictive while others are highly addictive. So why couldn't still other substances (which fall below the normal threshold of what we consider addiction) also demonstrate addictive tendencies?

I could be completely wrong, of course. I am no more skilled in biochemistry and biomechanical functions than I am qualified to write a diet book. Nevertheless, given the limited information I have, my conclusions seem logical to me. Maybe they do to you too. I can see no other explanation for insane eating behavior patterns—patterns which otherwise defy all logic.

If you want some evidence of these patterns, let's examine a case study. Around this same time in our story, there were three people: Stephanie, Sam, and Yours Truly.* We worked in the same office. One of our favorite lunchtime activities happened to be hitting the All You Can Eat Buffet. Was there ever a more telling icon of American culture? Where else could you find a pile of food capable of feeding a small village for a week for just $5.99 plus tax? Our goal was to search out as many buffets as we could (not all in one day) and to rate them according to the Three Vs: Volume, Variety, and Value.

We called our trio "The Snouts" and believed it was our destiny to write up a Buffet Review column in the local newspaper. Our trademark would have been the coveted "Three Snouts Up!" award—the highest rating any buffet proprietor could hope to achieve from three such renowned aficionados. Unfortunately, we didn't exactly have a large number of viable eating establishments in our area. Our column never saw the light of day and we never actually went to a buffet that wasn't either "pizza" or "Chinese."

When it was high time for another outing, we would carefully lay out our plan of attack through a complex series of signals. Specifically, one of us would ask, "Are you two hungry?" and the other two would say, "Yep. Let's go."

I don't ever recall any restaurant outright failing the three volume, variety, and value tests. Occasionally, a pizza place might not have enough of the right kinds of pies set out,

* Not their real names.

but more often than not, we were always satisfied. But to be honest, "satisfied" isn't the right term at all. *Satisfied* is what one would feel after leaving an All You *Care* To Eat buffet. We, on the other hand, were in the All You *Can* Eat mindset. We ate as if we'd paid $200 for lunch. We ate as if someone told us a meteor was heading to Earth and we only had twelve minutes to live. Invariably we could barely move by the meal's end. Worse, when we returned to work, we were completely worthless. We sat at our desks, bloated and tired and miserable. And for what? What purpose did it serve? Even if we actually had twelve minutes to live, why elect to spend them so uncomfortable and semi-comatose?

The answer is because it's *really* hard to keep seven billion billion billion atoms under control all at the same time. But I never thought of it that way at the time. I just thought I was worthless and weak.

So, where was I? Oh yeah—I was gaining weight. Try not to let me get off on tangents like that. You'll never know where I might end up. Anyway, we left off at 219.5 pounds. You'll be completely unsurprised to find out that only three months later, I'd gained even more weight. On April 17, 1995, the scale audibly chuckled as it displayed 221.0. I wrote:

> Ugh. Well, it was bound to happen. I broke into the 220s this morning. It was a bad weekend, food-wise. It was Easter so that meant a lot of candy.

Needless to say, this triggered yet another Day One. I managed to lose ten pounds in less than forty days, but bottomed out quickly. A few weeks later, I went on vacation, and sure enough, gained six back. ("Ugh. I didn't do so good." read that day's grammatically challenged entry.) After that, it was nothing but trampoline dieting as I vainly struggled to regain any sort of control. By mid-November (note: well before the Thanksgiving Curse) it just shot right up. I wrote:

> Man! Look at this! This has gotta stop! When I wrote the 224.5 entry I thought that would be a peak for a while. And here we are, moving right on up! This is unbelievable. I feel like I'm still in denial... what am I doing.
>
> I think I must have gone through some major metabolic change here or something. There's no other explanation for this sudden, recent rapid weight gain.

I was 227 pounds. But if you think it stops there, then think again. Remember, it's not even Thanksgiving yet. Here's what happened when we got back from our trip:

> Okay, this is it. I mean, this is REALLY it. I pigged out over the Thanksgiving holiday in Chicago. In fact, sometimes I think I almost went out of my way to eat more than usual (perhaps knowing that I'd be making some sort of resolution when it was over)

I was 229 and close to sheer panic. But before moving on, take a close look at what I wrote. What fascinates me now, looking back on all this, is this line: *in fact, sometimes I think I almost went out of my way to eat more than usual.* I didn't think anything of it at the time. And only now, looking back, do I realize this was the first time I experienced that particular feeling. (And I have felt it oh so many times since then.)

Most eating binges are of the type I described earlier. That is, your brain is offline but your body is in full feeding frenzy mode. But then there's this other strange sort of "lucid binging." You're not the mindless eating machine. In fact, quite the opposite is true. You're perfectly coherent and feeding your face for the same reason people climb mountains: *because it's there.* And not unlike mountain climbing, you feel like you're actually achieving a goal. Why is this?

The explanation is at hand. We don't even have to look any further than the next line for it: *perhaps knowing that I'd be making some sort of resolution when it was over.* In other words, given the full knowledge that I would be starting Yet Another Day One the following Monday, I'd somehow been given a license to binge. In a bizarre twist of rationale, I may have even been *trying* to pack on extra weight, for the sole reason of making the subsequent weight loss more dramatic. Who says sugar isn't mind-altering?

This new high was enough to drive me to diet during December. I don't think I'd ever done that before (or since, for that matter.) I actually managed to get down to nearly 220 just before Christmas. This isn't much of an accomplishment given those last fast pounds are the easiest to pull off again. And it's even less of an accomplishment considering they were nearly all back by New Year's Eve.

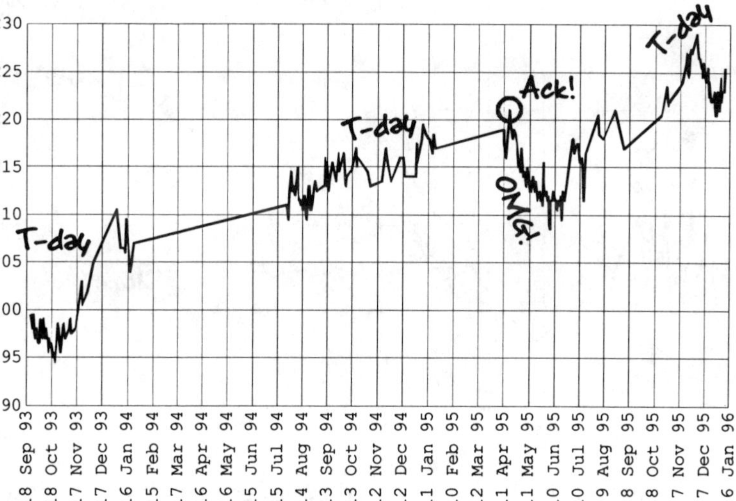

If at this point you're expecting the traditional New Year's diet to begin, you're going to be disappointed. It didn't happen this year. It was 1996 and the worst weight gain year ever for me. I was working a full-time day job while trying to run my own business in my so-called off hours. It was the first time in my life I'd ever worked hours like that: more than seventy a week, on average, for weeks and months on end. I spent all day sitting and working and eating. I was only one bad case of jaundice away from looking like a replica of Homer Simpson.

I had two sources of exercise: 1) walking down the stairs to my home office and 2) lifting food up to my face. Remarkably, I even went three months without stepping on a scale. I just didn't care any more. In June, I passed 230 for the first time. But I didn't write a thing about it. I have no idea now how I felt at the time, but I think the absence of an entry speaks for itself. The following October saw 234, yet I still didn't do anything about it. The holidays came as usual and on December 28, 1996, I peaked. This final chart tells the story best.

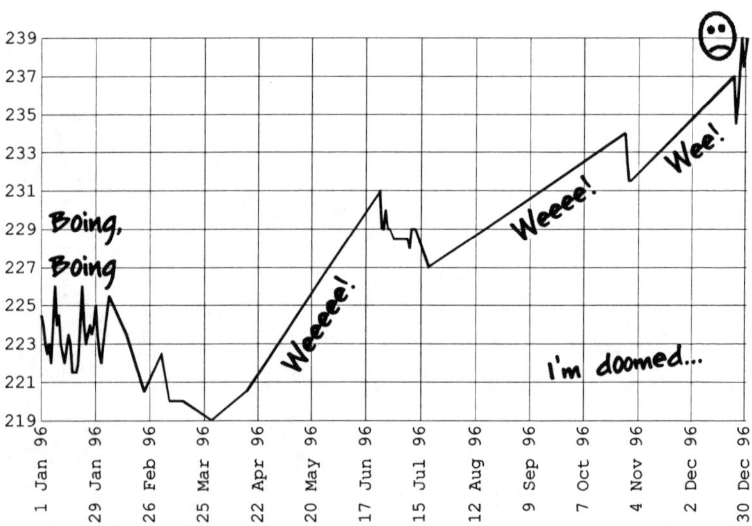

That was it. I *had* to do something now. Two hundred and thirty nine was the limit. There was absolutely, positively *no way* I was going to go into the 240s. But what was I to do? I'd already tried dieting and exercising on my own without lasting success. Was it finally time to try a more "official" approach? There certainly wasn't a shortage of roads to the Promised Land, as we saw in the previous chapter. But could any of them possibly work for me?

Chapter 6

Why Are We So Fat?

If you're in a hurry and just want me to answer the question right now, here goes: it's because we eat too much and don't move around enough. Period. There's no mystery or disagreement over about the basic facts. You may now move on to the next chapter. However, if you're a bit curious about how we arrived at this point (and you're not in *that* much of a hurry), then stick around. This could get interesting.

Defining "Overweight"

According to the American Obesity Association, about one third of all Americans are classified as obese. If you throw in the people who are simply overweight, the total doubles to two thirds. Even people at the upper end of the "normal" range could stand to lose a few pounds. Lump these folks in with the others and you have upwards of eighty percent of the population in desperate need of a carrot. Obviously, we have a problem. It's equally obvious that the ten billion weight loss solutions already out there aren't solving a dang thing.

Whether you're classified as overweight or obese depends on your BMI, or "Body Mass Index." This figure is calculated by taking the number of pumpkin pies you eat in a year and multiplying it by the number of tubs of movie popcorn you eat, squared. Take me as an example. I generally eat seven pumpkin pies a year and twenty-four tubs of popcorn. That gives me a BMI of 583. This legally classifies me as "rotund" and makes me eligible for life insurance benefits at a monthly premium equal to my BMI times two, divided by my height in meters.

Wait a minute. This doesn't sound right. I think I need to hire a new fact-checker. Hang on a sec...

Okay, I got it. (Sorry about that.) The Body Mass Index is a simple relationship between weight and height. It's expressed as either weight divided by height squared (metric units) or weight divided by height squared times 703 (English units). Once you have this number, you end up in one of these categories:

- **Underweight**: less than 18.5
- **Normal or Ideal**: from 18.5 to 24.9
- **Overweight**: from 25.0 to 29.9
- **Obese**: from 30.0 to 39.9
- **Morbidly Obese or Rock-hard Bodybuilder**: 40 +

If you want to calculate your own index, you can plug your numbers into one of the above formulas or you can do a Google search and find one of about ten thousand BMI calculators already out there. This is what I've just tried and have come up with a (current) BMI of 31.2.*

---

*So it's official. I'm obese. The funny thing is I don't feel like it. I mean, sure, I could clearly stand to lose a few pounds, but *obese*? That simply doesn't seem right. Maybe it's just that word—too many negative connotations.

I also discovered the low end of the ideal weight range for someone my height is 130 pounds. Can you believe that? Yeah, maybe if I was fourteen. But an actual five foot eleven adult human male weighing 130 pounds? That just doesn't seem right.

I'm not alone. We're large. There's no doubt about it. The United States has always prided itself on being an innovative nation. After all, this is the country that came up with both the light bulb *and* Barney the Dinosaur—hardly trivial accomplishments. But somewhere along the way, we pioneered the concept of "bigger is better" too. Thinking small just isn't the American Way, and food is another aspect of this mindset.

However, just as the light bulb and Barney have found their way across the globe, the United States is no longer an exclusive haven of adipose tissue. Obesity follows industrialization like stink follows a skunk. According to the World Health Organization, seventy-five percent of women over the age of thirty are overweight in countries such as Egypt, South Africa, Turkey and Mexico. The same is true of men in Greece, Germany, New Zealand and the United Kingdom. The scale tops out in the Western Pacific islands of Nauru and Tonga where nine of every ten adults is overweight. I wonder if that tenth person feels like a social outcast.

Some of these countries accomplish these feats all on their own. Others have our help. You can find Coca-Cola in over two hundred countries. McDonald's logs half of its receipts outside the United States and they're just two of an untold number of companies contributing to the world's waistline.

The Physiological Component

To help understand the cause of all this, let's travel back in time to see how humans made a living tens of thousands of years ago. Try to imagine early civilization: a time where technology was no more advanced than spears and hand-axes. People lived in small groups and spent most of their time simply surviving. The acts of hunting, gathering, and preparing food consumed most of their waking hours. There are two extremely important points to note here:

- Hunting and gathering expends a lot of energy.
- They weren't hunting and gathering potato chips.

As you can see, "eating right and exercising" isn't some twentieth century fad—it's how we were intended to function. Even more importantly, this lifestyle didn't exactly lend itself to overeating. Quite the opposite, actually. The human body spent many thousands of years adapting to a scarcity of food, and when you're trying to survive, it's not in your best long-term interest to die of starvation. The body needed some sort of mechanism to prevent this and nature happily obliged by giving men guts and women butts. Here's how it works.

The cell is the smallest structural and functional unit of the body. They are truly amazing things. A full discussion of them would require an entire shelf of books, so I won't go into any more detail than this: they're small, they require energy, and they're what make you *you*. Turn them off or start a feud between them and you cease to exist. It's as simple as that.

From their point of view, our bodies must be inconceivably gigantic machines. It takes about one hundred trillion of them just to make *one* of us.* As you can imagine, a lot of fuel is required to keep them all fed. The fuel they use is glucose. This is why you eat. It's not because you're hungry, or happy, or sad, or on vacation, or even bored. You eat to keep your one hundred trillion little buddies going, and they have lots of ways of making you get their glucose for them.

Their fuel comes from two basic sources: intake and reserves, with the preference *greatly* given to intake. Glucose is broken down from carbohydrates most easily, but your body can get it out of proteins and fats if it absolutely has to. Once broken down into glucose, the fuel "hits the highway" so to speak and enters your bloodstream. There it would circulate forever if not for the help of a small but extraordinary polypeptide hormone called insulin.

---

* Stack them one on top of another and you could make 2.6 trips to the moon. (It's true. I did it once.) Or consider this: if each cell were the size of a basketball, you could fill a box seven miles to a side.

Insulin is responsible for more things than I could ever hope to write about—here or anywhere else. What's important to us here is that insulin is what negotiates with your cells to let the glucose in. The cells burn what they need, the rest is sent to long-term storage. In fact, it is this very storage problem that brings us all together today.

Anyway, back to our ancestors. Where were we? Oh yeah, hunting for meat and gathering plants—two things which meant moving around a lot. Because of the scarcity of food, you never, ever had cave-mothers telling their cave-children "Eat your food! There are starving people in Thugronda!" Quite the opposite. When food was available, you *ate* it—no questions asked. The body had no idea when the next meal was coming, so it sent very strong signals: "eat while you can and as much as you can." And since "as much as you can" was very, very rarely "too much" this wasn't a bad system.

This is how we lived for tens of thousands of years. Life was purely about survival. It was primitive and repetitive.* Then one day, out of the blue, we decided we needed to invent agriculture. I can only assume we were tired of seeing the countryside and staying fit and trim. There are many theories about this important transition, everything from decreasing animal populations to discovering that plants could be grown on purpose. For whatever reason, people began growing more and gathering less. This meant we didn't move around as much and a larger percentage of our diets came from carbohydrates—a move that would cost American consumers billions of dollars in the late twentieth century.

The increase in carbs at the dawn of agriculture did not initially make people fat. This is because ancient carbs were in the form of small dried pebbles plucked from plants—a far cry from the modern French fry. Further, they weren't being

---

* It's a comfort to know we've advanced to the point where we now spend the bulk of our day sitting in office cubicles.

eaten to excess. These were whole grains, full of good stuff and slowly digested. The body had no trouble with it. Then a funny thing happened on the way to the fat farm: technology.

The Technological Component

It's not a stretch to see that on certain days, our ancestors' basic survival needs might be met in less time than on other days. Whether due to optimal conditions, sheer luck, or good karma, they might occasionally find themselves with a little extra time. Some may have spent the time down at the corner sports bar but others perhaps would have used it to improve tools. It's then conceivable that the new tools meant that the next day they might have had even *more* time. Thus, the technology spiral begins: time begets progress and progress begets time. Most inventions improve a process and in many cases, improvements focus on efficiency. When a process becomes more efficient, you'll either spend *less* time getting an equal output or spend an equal time getting *more* output.

This phenomenon then creates the concept of a *job*. (Gee, thanks, ancestors!) If a family produces ten times the amount of food as before, they are now no longer able to consume it by themselves. They now have the ability to provide for others in their community. It then follows that if others can have their food requirements satisfied by this family, they no longer have to spend their time on it. They're now freed up to do other things: presumably, producing goods and services in exchange for the food.

Fast forward some thousands of years, to the point where production changes from a small, family-owned endeavor into an industry all unto itself. As the industry grows, efficiency is paramount. Food is distributed through vast networks—much larger than anything society ever before imagined. The size of the distribution networks suddenly makes food preservation an issue. As the system grows ever larger, selling more food becomes a necessity *solely to support the infrastructure*. In other words, it's no longer about "I have some food, you need some food, so let's trade." It's about "I have an enterprise I must maintain, and I'll do anything to maintain it—including lying through advertising and using cheapo ingredients." Now it's all finally coming together:

1. Humans grew up hunting and gathering.
2. We then settled down to grow our own plants.
3. Settling down led to jobs.
4. Jobs led to industries.
5. Industries eventually put money first.
6. Money first means your health comes second.

The Hormonal Component

The impact of various foods on blood sugar levels is rated by something called the glycemic index. Foods high on the index, such as chocolate bars and white bread, cause blood sugar levels shoot up. Foods low on the index, like turkey or cheese, have little or no affect on blood sugar.

When high glycemic foods hit your system, not only do blood sugar levels spike quickly, they also drop quickly soon after. The spike triggers the pancreas to release insulin to take care of the situation. Unfortunately, this can leave too much insulin floating around after it's finished. Ironically, the body now cries out, "Sugar levels too low!"

In response to this cry, two things happen. First, this condition forces a follow-up wave of hormones to help rebalance the system. If all goes well, the liver releases glucose back into the bloodstream and everything eventually levels out. Second, this condition sends out hunger signals. After all, the quickest gosh darn way to get your blood sugar levels back up is by eating more sugar. That's right! In response to eating a big plate of mashed potatoes and gravy, about an hour or so later, your body yells out, "I'm hungry!" Think about the warped logic here. In a panic response to an out-of-whack system, your body demands an action that will only perpetuate the out-of-whackness. Isn't the first rule of holes, "When you're in one, stop digging"?

I'm amazed that the body can handle this kind of abuse for as long as it does. But it can't do it forever. Let's say you hit the local fast food joint for the twenty thousandth time. You order the regular burger, fries, and a soda. You flood your system with vast amounts of glucose-rich foods. Again. The pancreas releases insulin. Again. The insulin carries the glucose to the cells, and the cells at last protest, "You have *got* to be kidding me. You were *just* here an hour ago." Then the cells across the hall pipe in, "And an hour before that, too! Now bugger off!" Dejected, the poor insulin continues to drag the glucose around door to door, only to have door after door slammed in its face. Since the glucose can't leave the bloodstream, the body continues to send out the signal, "Hey, blood sugar levels are too high. Better send more insulin out."

Now you're in trouble. Welcome to insulin resistance. Next stop, diabetes. Thanks to your tireless efforts, you broke your own body's ability to regulate its fueling system.

Obviously, this is completely the fault of that fast food restaurant, right? It's certainly not *your* fault. They never told you that French fries would break your pancreas. Something *that* important would be in big red letters across the Super Combo Menu, wouldn't it? You'd better go file that lawsuit now, before someone discovers the truth.

For the record, it's not their fault. And all sarcasm aside, it's not really your fault either. Although I first discussed this in terms of addiction back on page 45, now that we've had our history and physiology lessons, things should be a bit clearer. To summarize, the human body grew up on food in scarce supply. The body, for reasons of pure survival—*instinct,* if you will—eats as much food as it can get, knowing the next meal could be days away. For these same reasons, it prefers high-energy foods, which the body craves—nay, *demands*—above all others. Then on the rare occasions it gets too much food, it can store it as fat for use later on.

Now take this human out of the ideal environment where food is scarce and exercise is plentiful. Just for fun—even as a sick, twisted joke—let's put this human in an environment where food is never more than a few yards away and exercise is something that only happens between the car and the elevator. Suddenly your innate survival skills are working against you in a way Mother Nature never foresaw. We were *never* prepared for this. We aren't *supposed* to have pie holes, because we were never meant to have pie. We've created a world around us that couldn't be more wrong for our physical well-being. And the armchair quarterbacks think you have no willpower!

Believe it or not, not everybody is overweight. Somehow, a certain percentage of individuals have figured out a way to outsmart this system I've just described. They either make better food choices or exercise more, or both. Or perhaps they've simply been blessed with hormones and a metabolic engine that burns fuel more efficiently than the rest of us do. It's our job to find these people and make them eat a lot of cookies and ice cream, because they're really starting to make the rest of us look bad.

If some of these people remain thin thanks to a sound and balanced hormonal system, then it only logically follows that the rest of us ended up with a not-so-good system. There are definitely people for whom eating right and exercising alone doesn't work. Worse, there are those for whom eating right and exercising isn't even an option. They're apparently preprogrammed to eat and eat and eat. And once that takes over, exercising isn't even a remote possibility.

Every so often, you'll see their stories on television. They weigh anywhere between 600 and 800 pounds. They're bedridden and miserable. Yet they continue to eat. "Show a little willpower, fatso!" That's what conventional wisdom would shout at them. Conventional wisdom thinks these people have no one to blame but themselves. Conventional wisdom can't understand why they just won't go on a diet. Conventional wisdom isn't very bright sometimes.

Since you've gotten this far in the book, you already know what I'm going to say. I'll argue to my dying breath that this is not a failure of willpower. Whatever regulating mechanism normally exists, they simply don't have it. They'll consume upwards of 30,000 calories a day because their body has the "feed me" signal and no corresponding "I'm full" signal. The hormone responsible for the former is ghrelin. Cells in the stomach lining produce it and it is responsible for stimulating appetite at appropriate times. The complimentary hormone controlling the latter is leptin and it manages appetite and metabolism, among other things. It should be obvious that if the body is producing one hormone and not the other, you'll have a really bad situation on your hands.

I feel terrible for these people—and even more so because from the outside it *seems* like it should be such a simple thing to fix. "Just eat less! You'll lose weight! Show a little willpower!" There goes that stupid conventional wisdom again, spouting off like an idiot.

Personally, I don't believe nature gives us simple on/off switches. While I have no scientific evidence to back this up, I simply don't believe a person either does or doesn't have the proper levels of ghrelin and leptin. It just seems far more likely it would fall along a continuum. Towards the left, and you keep very thin. Towards the right, and you end up in a medical journal. Most of us are in the middle. Does that make sense? It does to me and I'm ever anxious to learn more.

The Genetic Component

I have two sisters, Beth and Jennifer.* They are identical twins, but when it comes to weight struggles, the three of us may as well be triplets. Old family photos reveal a long line of weight issues. In spite of that, the three of us certainly

---

* Not their real names. Their real names are Jennifer and Beth.

started out skinny enough. Even at the age of thirteen, I remained your textbook ninety-eight pound weakling. My dad would talk about "the Hills gut" and declare (with an air of relief in his voice) that I was probably going to escape the fate that befell all those before me. I'd say things even looked hopeful for Beth and Jenn too for a good, long while. Not one of us showed any signs of uncontrolled expansion.

A common argument in many fields of human study is "nature versus nurture." That is to say, does a condition arise inherently due to your genetic makeup or is it introduced through certain behavior patterns?

It's easy to declare we're fat due to involuntary biological signals. ("Nature!") However, it's just as easy to declare it's because we never learned to eat right. ("Nurture!")

I'm not a scientist, and so I don't really care which one is the right answer. All I know is that I started out skinny and now I'm not. I looked perfectly fine when I was thirteen. Eight years later, I wasn't. I don't think my DNA changed all that much in that time. I do know that during that time I ate about four hundred bowls of Cap'n Crunch and drank about six hundred Big Gulps from 7-11. But then again, I had more than one friend at the time with similar eating patterns, and they didn't gain weight the way my sisters and I did.

Cleaning the garage one day, I happened to find both my high school and college graduation photos. By some chance, they were taken from nearly the exact same angle and so served as a good comparison. The change was stunning. It's amazing what four years of all-night studying fueled by two hundred gallons of soda pop can do.

Anyway, it all boils down to this: no matter what factors are working against you, it's important to believe that you still have some say in the matter. Maybe your family is overweight. Maybe your species is overweight. Maybe you're simply a sucker for chips and dip. Who cares. If you think your "I'm Full" signal is only slightly out of whack, try to rid yourself of your negative triggers. That may be just enough to get you back on your feet. If your signal is completely out of whack, seek professional help. There's nothing wrong with asking for help.

And if none of that works, well, at least maybe you'll get to be on television one day.

The Pleasure Component

In some ways, I think the easiest answer to "Why are we so fat?" is summed up with, "Because we love food!" There's no doubt that eating can be a most pleasurable experience and we are, as a rule, predisposed to repeat pleasurable experiences as often as possible.

My own ideal diet would be made up from the four basic food groups: Italian, Mexican, Chinese, and Cheeseburgers. While I would be hard-pressed to pick a favorite, I can say in all confidence that I could eat one big, juicy cheeseburger every day for one year and not get tired of it. (I may alternate sides between onion rings and French fries just for variety, but never doubt they're only there to serve the sandwich.)

Wait. Did I say, "Because we love food?" I really meant, "Because we love food *and* because there's a food industry all too willing to take advantage of it." Here's how that industry took advantage of me and my adoration of the aforementioned cheeseburger.

One innocent day a coupon showed up in the newspaper for a free Monster Burger* from Hardee's. The coupon claimed how much larger it was than a Whopper or a Big Mac (which honestly isn't saying much) and invited you to try one on the house (the first one's always free, as taught in Drug Dealing 101). I duly informed The Snouts, and we all agreed we were up for the taste test. So with coupons in hand, the three of us headed out to see what all the fuss was about.

---

* This was the original Monster Burger in 1996. It is definitely not the same as the Monster Thickburger introduced in 2004.

Frankly, we were a bit disappointed. It was only marginally larger than the King and the Clown's offerings. We inhaled them with little effort and decided we needed to seek out an even bigger burger. Thus, the Challenge was born.

We racked our brains for all of three seconds before deciding on our next stop. We made a beeline to Wendy's (no, not the same day) to order us up a trio of Triples. Certainly, a burger with three quarter-pound patties would trump the wimpy "Monster" Burger. Sam got up to the counter first and requested the first triple. Stephanie was next. By the time I ordered mine, the folks working in back were already peering out curiously to see who (or what) was at the counter.

This clearly wasn't normal lunchtime behavior.

They clearly had never met The Snouts.

We carried our laden trays to the dining room where we plopped ourselves down and immediately set on our burgers like hyenas on a kill. They were good, juicy and big—but not quite big enough. We had to move on.

We caught wind that a local bar served a full one-pound burger made up of three one-third pound patties. There was no arguing that this was the next stop in our Quest.

On the chosen day, we drove to the bar. We entered a smoky room and found a table. We needed no menus; we were here for one reason only. The waitress arrived and took our heavy order, unfazed. We sat in rapt anticipation, engaging in mindless small talk only to pass the minutes until our feast arrived. Before long, the burgers were set before us and we pounced. They were singularly perfect. To this day, I'm not sure I've had better. They were juicy, but not greasy. They were cooked to perfection. This was the work of artists.

You'd think that'd be enough for us, wouldn't you? Well, you'd be wrong. In spite of cheeseburger perfection, we began discussing where our mission might lead us next. Someone had heard of a truck stop east of town that served a four-pound burger. The meat made up two of the four pounds, the bun and toppings made up the rest. We had no choice. We had to find and eat this burger.

Four of us went on this particular trip and we ordered two of the behemoths between us. This meant nearly twice the total volume of the last burger, per person. Once again, we placed our plus-sized order without menus. As we waited, the talk turned to the burger preparation. Exactly how long would it take to cook a single two-pound patty? We discussed the various techniques and stratagems that might solve this particular problem. The more we discussed it, the more we began to wonder if it might be an hour or more before our food arrived.

Surprisingly, we didn't wait long at all. Every head in the dining room turned toward us as the waitress delivered the majestic mounds of meat to our eager table. We quickly sliced each burger down the middle and divided the four halves between us. Upon taking our first bites, we realized why they arrived so quickly.

"I think they're pre-cooked," one of us noted.

"I think you're right," the rest of us agreed.

They were dry and for the most part quite unsatisfying. This was, of course, a terrible letdown considering, 1) how unearthly the previous burger was, and 2) this was undoubtedly the end of our big burger trek. If I recall correctly, we didn't even finish them. We paid our bill and rejoined the world of normal, quarter pound hamburgers.

A good decade or more has passed since then but I don't think a quest like this is every truly over. I still keep one eye peeled for the next big burger. My guess is I'll have to look no further than Denny's Beer Barrel Pub in Clearfield, Pennsylvania. They serve burgers in the following denominations: two pounds, three pounds, six pounds, fifteen pounds, and—hold on to your diapers—*fifty* pounds. That's right! For just $179.95 (and twenty-four hours notice), you and six dozen or more of your closest friends can partake in one cow on a bun.

Okay, so why are we so fat again?

Chapter 7

The History of Dieting

Recent archeological findings suggest that eating began around 35,000 years ago. Before that, humans simply didn't eat at all. The reason was obvious: there just wasn't any time to eat, what with having to spend most of the day avoiding Sleestaks and marauding dinosaurs. If you reached your eighteenth birthday, you were officially considered a senior citizen and eligible for clan retirement benefits. Sure, people didn't last very long back then, but they were, as a rule, remarkably fit and trim.

The evidence for the dawn of eating comes from a large, flat stone recently unearthed during an excavation in Eastern Europe. What at first looked like a featureless surface was eventually shown to contain faint inscriptions. Upon close examination, linguistics experts were able to discern the following writings:

> May 12, 33,142 B.C. We just killed off the last dinosaur a few days ago. No one's seen a Sleestak for months. We're kind of bored now. Bogg planted some seeds he found over by those rocks.

> July 21, 33,142 B.C. Bogg's seeds sprouted some time ago and are growing into tall plants. No idea what they are. And we're still bored. What we wouldn't give for cable television right about now.

> October 2, 33,142 B.C. Seeds turned into some nice, yellow sweet corn. Not knowing what else to do with it, we put it in our mouths, chewed it up, and swallowed it. Not bad. Think we'll try again next year.

Aside from the discovery that English is far older than anyone had imagined, the scientific community was stunned by the date that eating began. (Before this finding, it was a widely accepted fact that eating didn't begin until April 14 of the following year.)

The following year Bogg & Crew did plant more seeds and grew more corn. Their new "growing and harvesting" routine started a trend that quickly spread to neighboring communities. As food supplies grew, so did their bodies. It didn't take long before they realized something had to be done.

The Dr. Ayla Diet

This was the world's first diet, created by a Cro-Magnon physician named Ayla. For those readers unfamiliar with her, she was not only a great doctor but also a highly prolific inventor, responsible for the introduction of just about everything from flint-and-steel to plasma television screens. As proto-Europeans stuffed themselves silly with sweet corn, they started noticing stone wheels growing around their midsections. Ayla correctly surmised that this heretofore-unknown malady was a direct result of over-eating, and thus prescribed a strict regimen of "no more than two ears a day." For those that could adhere to this diet, the results were immediate. Cave-elder Tharg recounts his personal experience. "I used to eat as much corn as I could get: upwards of six or seven ears a day. Often, we would milk animals, separate the cream from the milk and churn it. The resulting substance was *to die for* when spread all over the corn. But my growing stone wheel soon got in the way of ordinary activities and I knew I had to do something. Dr. Ayla's Diet was the ticket! I look and feel as good now at 18 as I did when I was 16! Thanks Dr. Ayla!"

Cleopatrasize

Cleopatra's renowned beauty did not come easy. It is a little known historical truth that she did, in fact, struggle with her weight most of her life. While she tried every diet known to Egypt, she found little success. What finally worked turned out to be good, old-fashioned exercise.

It all began one restless night. Unable to sleep, she demanded entertainment. However, due to the hour, the usual performers were nowhere to be found. But as fate would have it, one person was available. He seemed to be promoting some sort of exercise system. He began by describing the benefits of his program then summoned at least two dozen followers, each of them mimicking his every move. Cleopatra was at once enthralled. They seemed to be performing Greek boxing mixed with martial art movements from the Far East. They were puffing and sweating a great deal, but all looked exceedingly happy in spite of it. Every once in a while one would break off from the rest of the group and tell his or her personal story of how this program changed his or her life.

Cleopatra was moved. She wasted no time in paying the 29.95 denarii for the instructions and set right to work. The frenzied dance-like movements, the kicks, the punches—they all seemed to melt the pounds away. It wasn't long before she decided she needed to get the word out too. She soon began promoting it as *Cleopatrasize*. She gave local performances, wrote several scrolls on the topic, and quickly became a sensation. Word spread to Rome where Mark Antony, himself needing a bit of a workout, traveled to Egypt to see this craze.

They met, fell in love, and lost at least seven or eight more pounds before Rome became angered with Antony's weight loss. Octavian sent a fleet of ships to attack Egypt. Antony and Cleopatra, seeing the invincible Roman armada approach, decided they needed one more workout before fighting. Unfortunately, they both died from last minute, over-zealous Cleopatrasizing. Let that be a lesson to us all.

The Camelot Diet

In his later years, as King Arthur started to pack on the pounds, he asked Merlin for dieting advice. Merlin studied the problem and worked on it for six months before coming up with a solution. It worked like a charm. In fact, it *was* a charm, but that didn't stop people from wanting a part of it. Once they saw their new, svelte king prancing about the countryside, the "Camelot Diet" (as it immediately came to be called) was an instant hit. In fact, it's generally regarded as the very first diet that went on to become a national craze. Merlin was ultimately forced to write a book. Scribes enlisted at monasteries churned out copies at upwards of two dozen per year: an unprecedented best-seller. People across the country paid a ha'penny per copy. Gross receipts reached nearly half a crown within the first year of publication. Unfortunately, no one but Merlin was actually able to get it to work, but that didn't stop people from trying. Some things never change.

The Renaissance Diet

As Europe emerged from the dark ages, the newly enlightened population suddenly remembered it liked to eat. Perhaps in defiance of earlier hard times, over-eating became fashionable. Women everywhere adopted the *Rubenesque* look, named after Flemish painter Peter Paul Rubens, who himself went on to create the lovable Pee-wee Herman character.

Alas! Fashions change faster than the weather, and it wasn't long before slimming was back in. The newly revived weight loss craze was nowhere more popular than in England, where it became a group activity. Essentially an entire village would gather on weekends to work out together. Participants donned special exercise clothing (generally dressing as their favorite characters from *Monty Python and the Holy Grail* or *The Lord of the Rings*) to re-enact sword fights and hold jousting tournaments. One would also find the expected mix of minstrels and troubadours, jesters and jugglers. It was all good fun and not uncommon for participants to lose one or two stone in their first two months of working out.

The New World Diet

Once Europeans finally learned how to stay alive in the New World, sure enough, some grew overweight. The New World diet was fashioned after the great harvest feast of 1621. This ultra-strict diet included portions of turkey, stuffing, mashed potatoes, yams, green bean casserole, and cranberry sauce. These foods were to be taken almost daily. It was difficult to tell at first if the diet had any affect, as the test subjects pretty much slept all the time. For the brief periods where they were awake, they were generally found to have *gained* weight, much to the dismay of early New World dieticians.

"We don't understand," the early dieticians said in a press conference. "The first tyme we ate like this, there was not a single incident of corpulence among us. We thoughte unquestionably that by reintroducing these foods, it would certainly bring corpulent persons in-line with 1621 demographics." They concluded the press conference by stating they needed "more researche." The last record we have on this diet shows that in a last-ditch effort to boost its effectiveness, they added "pumpkin pie and whippéd creame" to the regimen.

The Industrial Diet

As Western society shifted emphasis from agriculture to industry, changes in eating patterns were inevitable—and so followed dieting. Several diets came and went but only one from this period takes its place in the annals of our dietary history: the Industrial Diet. On this plan, persons who wished to lose weight were sent to sweatshops to work 98 hours per week. Weight loss was guaranteed. Additionally, this is the only diet in history where dieters actually earned money for dieting. Although wages were only about seventy-five cents a week, that was better than nothing. After just three months, the typical subject had lost about thirty pounds and the will to live. But he'd also earned enough money to buy a second-hand horse, which he promptly ate.

The Regular Diet

Most of us grew up with this diet. It invariably takes the shape of some regular geometric object and recommends you to eat some foods more than others. The proportions change in response to food industry lobbying, so it's hard to tell what's good for you at any given moment.

The government spends millions of dollars attempting to educate us on the meaning of the various shapes and colors. They understand the importance of everyone learning the Regular Diet. They send posters to schools, which are prominently displayed next to the soda and snack machines. Every child thus learns the importance of good nutrition whilst grabbing eighty-seven grams of excess fats and carbohydrates from Vend-O-Land. Adults learn about the Regular Diet from food packages. Bread packages tell you how important grain is. Dairy packages stress the importance of udder products.

In the end, what the Regular Diet usually represents is depravity and suffering. Cut out the stuff you most like to eat, and by golly, you're gonna lose the weight. How can you fail?

The Fad Diet

Since the Regular Diet apparently wasn't making anyone bucket loads of money, the Fad Diet was created. The primary goal of the diet is to get ten million people to buy the book. The primary goal of the book is to get you, the consumer, to read six pages, try two recipes, then shelve it while you go shopping for The Next Fad Diet Book.

This is a wonderful approach which has earned countless authors untold millions of dollars. A solid one-half percent of Fad Diet users have found successful, long-term weight loss using these programs. The other ninety-nine and a half percent are waiting for the Next Book to ship from Amazon.com.

The Women's Magazine Diet

To the untrained eye, the Women's Magazine Diet looks strikingly similar to the Fad Diet. However, a closer look will reveal important differences. This diet routinely begins with an article called **THE TRUTH ABOUT THE FAD DIET**. This in-depth piece of journalism exposes the lies you were taught by the Fad Diet's author. Invariably, the article tells you that what you *thought* made you thin actually makes you fat and vice versa. It trots out a semi-scientific study involving two groups of people. As expected, the group on *your* diet lost some weight but quickly gained it all back (and then some). Worse, the weight they *did* lose was all water and muscle tissue, so you can plainly see how stupid you were for trying that diet.

Luckily, they know how to save you from your dilemma—without any dieting! First, cut calories by making minor meal replacements. ("Swap your daily morning triple chocomocha frappelatte for a cup of green tea!") Second, burn calories with pseudo-exercises. ("Forget your remote. Walk to the TV!") By making 117 simple changes such as these to your daily lifestyle, you can lose ten pounds a year forever.

Don't worry if you missed the most recent "truth about" issue of your favorite women's magazine, they'll run another one just like it next month. You'll find it listed on the cover of every single issue, just to the left of the enormous chocolate cake photo. (**OUR "DECADENT DOZEN" DESSERT RECIPES**.)

Chapter 8

Mixed Messages

As I've already mentioned, we already know the key to weight loss. We don't have to play dumb. We don't have to rely on "experts" to tell us the right thing to do. We have to get up and move around a little more. We have to resist the urges to stuff ourselves silly. Simple? Yes. Easy? Not in the least bit.

And if things weren't hard enough, we are further hindered by a non-stop barrage of messages coming at us from every direction at once. It's easy to get confused. Even the most closely held truths could be doubted in the face of constant contradiction. And constant contradiction is essentially what we live with day in and day out.

It's not always easy to distinguish truth from fiction; or truth from half-truths; or truth from advertising; or even truth from outright dishonesty. But the most difficult task is distinguishing truth from truth. This is at the very heart of the mixed messages we receive day in and day out.

Take a look at Subway. Oh, what a gold mine they found in Jared Fogle. Unless you've been living in a Y2K survival shelter for the last several years, you know that Jared is *the man*.

At twenty years old, he found himself tipping the scales at 425 lbs. Deciding that enough was enough, he put himself on a 1,000 calorie a day diet. The plan? Two trips a day to the Subway shop next to his apartment. He stuck to turkey and veggie sandwiches, diet soft drinks, and, sure enough, the weight came off. After a time, he began walking a mile and a half a day and ultimately lost 245 pounds.

Word eventually found its way to Subway who began using Jared and his story to promote their lower-calorie offerings. And this is where it becomes difficult to separate truth from truth. What's really going on in these commercials? Each one typically presents a smiling, happy, thin Jared telling us how wonderful Subway is and how much McDonald's sucks. The implication, as near as I can tell, is that if you eat at Subway you are guaranteed to lose weight. If you eat at McDonald's, you will die.

Hmmm...this is a great example of how two truths can be added together to make something extremely misleading. Mr. Fogle did dine regularly at Subway while losing 245 pounds. And yes, certain Subway offerings are healthier than certain McDonald's offerings. But they've taken these two facts and rolled them into something misleading: eat at Subway for guaranteed good health. Eat elsewhere at your own peril.

And what's the average person going to do with this powerful message? They're probably going to drive to Subway, and order themselves up a distinctly non-diet, twelve-inch Steak & Cheese. It doesn't matter that the fine print says only certain sandwiches (with the good condiments removed) qualify as the healthful alternatives. The overriding message is, "Subway: Good; McDonald's: Bad." That's what sticks with the average person.

I mean, let's really think about Jared's diet. He consumed 1,000 calories a day (which is dramatically low for a six foot, two inch twenty year old male) and walked one and a half miles a day. I may be going out on a limb here, but it seems to me *that's* why he lost weight. It wasn't due to some Magical

Weight Loss Sandwiches. I mean, they're almost to the point now where they want you to think eating even *more* of them means even greater weight loss. Not too long ago, I saw one where Jared declared that the Big Mac has 33 grams of fat and Subway's twelve-inch chicken breast sandwich has only 10 grams of fat. He went on to proudly state that you could eat three of these sandwiches and still not match the fat of a Big Mac. Um, can we run the numbers on that?

	Calories	Fat	Carbs	Protein
Big Mac	600	33g	50g	25g
The 36" Chicken	1,980	30g	270g	114g

Is it just me or did he just tell me it's better to eat 1,980 Subway calories over 600 McDonald's calories? This from the fast food chain who seems so relentlessly concerned about my health? Something smells fishy here, and it isn't the six-inch tuna on wheat.

Well, here's the bad news, kids. Subway's first priority is not your health. Subway's first priority is to stay in business. Subway is a for-profit company in a free market. I will not fault them for wanting to earn money: that's the point of every business. What slightly annoys me is how relentlessly they portray their offerings as "good" when in reality only *some* of their menu items fall into the famous "6 Grams of Fat or Less" category.

Case in point: I myself ate at Subway regularly for years. I went every Tuesday because it was double stamp day. (And let me tell you, I *hoarded* those stamps. I think I just enjoyed the *thought* of all those free sandwiches more than the sandwiches themselves.*) My sandwich of choice was the Cold Cut Combo and, being the Real Man that I am, always ordered the

*Alas, they killed the stamp program but fortunately gave me enough heads up before my hard-earned stamps expired. I ate free-of-charge, about once a week, for about three months.

foot long.* Once properly decorated, the sandwich alone was easily pushing a thousand calories—never mind the chips and the (most certainly non-diet) drink. Ahhh...I still look back on it ever so fondly. Good times, good times.

While no longer a weekly event, I still make it to Subway from time to time. I like their food and it's a good, quick meal especially when you're on the go. But I'm not there because I'm trying to lose weight. I just want some food. But I can't help but worry about the poor folks lured in by "6 Grams or Less" who mess it up by ordering the wrong thing—yet still believe they've just eaten a Magical Weight Loss sandwich.

For another quick meal, our family also visits McDonald's occasionally. Laura enjoys their Premium Grilled Chicken sandwich. Why don't we make our own commercial and see how two of our favorite fast foods stack up against each other?

	Calories	Fat	Carbs	Protein
McDonald's Chicken	420	10g	51g	32g
Subway 12" Combo	1,040	92g	188g	84g

Wow. You don't see *that* on very many Subway commercials. Is it a fair comparison? Of course not. But neither are the real commercials. Anyone can carefully select the best item of one category and stack it up against the worst item of another. No actual lies take place, but these mixed messages have the potential to do as much harm as good.

Yes, Jared lost 245 pounds while eating at Subway. They are not about to let that go unnoticed. I fully expect they will continue promoting it for a good long while. Just don't read the fine print: "Individuals lost weight by exercising and eating a balanced, reduced-calorie diet. The SUBWAY® chain does not endorse the diet Jared created."

* With mayonnaise, of course. What self-respecting sandwich would be caught dead without mayonnaise on it? You might as well order pancakes without syrup.

While I may have issues with their marketing department, I must point out that Subway, to its credit, does put its money where its mouth is. They sponsor the American Heart Association through Heart Walks programs. Jared tours schools teaching the benefits of a healthy lifestyle. And lots of people in real life have indeed been inspired by Jared. Many, many pounds have been lost due to his high visibility. I can't find anything wrong with that.

Now let's turn our eyes to Subway's archenemy. (Or should I say, their *Golden Arch*enemy? Ha ha. I'm so witty.)

McDonald's sure takes a lot of heat for its position in the world. It's large. It's *very* large—a fact that positions it an obvious and ideal target for everything from environmental to health concerns. And, just like Subway, they're plenty guilty of sending mixed messages.

Look at a typical McDonald's commercial and what do you see? You see happy people. They are very happy. They are also exceedingly vibrant and healthy. This is no accident. This has been designed to attract you to their stores like moths to a flame. No one will visit a restaurant whose advertising is filled with depressed, slothful people, crawling in on hands and knees for their next scheduled feeding.

McDonald's is so huge that their advertising is almost irrelevant at this point. Most people will fall into one of these three categories:

1. Those who like McDonald's and will go there regardless of television ads.
2. Those who despise McDonald's and won't go there at gunpoint.
3. Those who would rather not go, but whose kids talk them into it anyway.

For those people in the first or third groups, the majority still order a burger, fries, and a Coke, or some slight variation thereof. "A burger, fries, and a Coke, you say! How evil! That's pure garbage. Never, *ever* put that stuff in your body." Thus speaks conventional wisdom again. But is it really so bad?

In 2004, filmmaker Morgan Spurlock released his movie *Super Size Me*. The premise was simple: eat at McDonald's every day, for thirty days, and see what happens. There were other rules, but the basic gist was just that: stick to a diet one hundred percent provided by the Big M Supper Club.

He began as a generally physically fit person and ended up dead. Just kidding. But to hear his doctor's tell it, you would have thought he was on death's door. And why think otherwise? In thirty days, he gained 24½ lbs. He experienced a wide variety of maladies ranging from depression to liver damage. He didn't feel good *at all*.

Wow. McDonald's really *is* evil! Maybe Jared was right!

Or here's a wild thought. Maybe he fared so poorly, not from eating at McDonald's per se, but from eating a high fat, high carb, low nutritional, 5,000-calorie per day diet. Yes, that's right. Five thousand calories per day.

I realize that he was only trying to demonstrate an already well-known point: that the food industry isn't primarily concerned with our health. They may show happy, healthy people in their commercials. They may proudly announce they have *some* healthful menu alternatives. But they're only there to make a fast buck and they'll do whatever it takes to get your dollars in their cash registers.

That said, you might be surprised to hear I'm siding with McDonald's on this one. I loved the movie and I agree with his basic message. But *man!* if you eat 5,000 calories a day of *anything* for weeks on end you're going to do some serious damage. Unless you're a triathlete preparing for the next Ironman, this is just plain wrong.

Is the food at McDonald's inherently bad? Well, as I've heard Alton Brown say, "There are no bad foods, just bad food habits." I don't believe the burger-fries-coke meal is any worse for you than the turkey-stuffing-potatoes meal you ate at your mom's last November or the lasagna-salad-cheesecake meal you had at your local, trendy *ristorante* on Saturday. It's all fat, carbs, and calories: your body doesn't care where it comes from. McDonald's bears the brunt of our ire, due to it being fast, cheap, and ubiquitous. Plus, neither your mom nor the local Italian place slams you with such in-your-face mixed-messages on a daily basis. But in the end, it's all the same to your body. So ignore the noise and don't feel bad if you enjoy a Big Mac *once in a while*. Just don't try to set any records.

The next issue is "not guilty by association." The key here is that if a company can strategically place its product in a healthful situation (or put one or two good things in it) then obviously the product is healthful too. Let me show you what I mean. Give me a minute or two while I run to the pantry.

[Insert *Jeopardy* theme here...]

Okay, here we go. Exhibit A is a box of Pop-Tarts. Ah ha, just as I thought! Right smack on the box front is a label that says it's a "Good Source of 7 Vitamins and Minerals." Huh? We're talking about a product that is over two hundred calories of flour, sugar, and fat. It has just ten percent of the recommended daily allowance for Vitamin A, Iron, Niacin, Thiamin, Vitamin B_6, Riboflavin, and Folic Acid. Ten percent! I might call this a *source* of vitamins and minerals. I wouldn't go all the way to *good*. Spinach is a good source of vitamins and minerals—not Pop-Tarts for heaven's sake.

Exhibit B is a can of Sour Cream and Onion flavored Pringles. I first need to go on record that I love these things. I love the Pringles like McAdams loves Gosling. And as for the sour cream and onion flavor? Wow. I'd buy sour cream and onion toothpaste if they made it. Anyway, this particular can of Pringles triumphantly declares that the product therein contains zero grams of trans fats. I'm not sure if you've noticed but *every* product nowadays is free of trans fats. I think my coconut-scented shampoo claims to be trans fat free. Never before have I seen such a sweeping change in so short a time. Not that I'm complaining: this is actually a good thing. But it has a dark side too: people are bound to make the same mistakes they did with fat free foods. They'll see nothing but the all-powerful "free" designation and go nuts with it. Case in point: KFC. Have you seen these commercials? Dads gone wild discovering that KFC is now trans fat free! Do you actually believe anyone was on a fried chicken hiatus solely due to trans fat concerns? Is fried chicken suddenly a calorie free food? Don't fall into that trap. Your body doesn't care how "free" it is. It's still counting calories even when you're not.

Exhibit C is a box of Honey Nut Cheerios. The happy bee flies around a huge red heart because Honey Nut Cheerios contains soluble fiber. The box proudly states, "Three grams of soluble fiber daily from whole grain oat foods, like Honey Nut Cheerios, in a diet low in saturated fat and cholesterol, may reduce the risk of heart disease. Honey Nut Cheerios has 0.75g per serving." So *if* you eat whole grain oats *and* reduce saturated fat and cholesterol in your diet you *may* reduce the risk of heart disease. The fine print tells the full story, yet the marketing message implies your only hope is this cereal. Does this mean it's bad? Not at all. There are certainly far worse things you can eat for breakfast. (Not to mention Honey Nut Cheerios are pretty darn tasty. I know I like them.) But you have to watch for the mixed messages. To get the recommended three grams of soluble fiber a day you would have to have four bowls of cereal, clocking in at about 600 calories. I'm sure there are better ways to get your soluble fiber. If we're lucky, they'll be sour cream and onion flavored too.

It's bad enough that corporate America sends mixed signals, but we also get them from the one place many of us turn to for help: the diet industry itself. Ironically, just about every program out there attempts to set itself apart by using the *exact same pitch*. "Confused by all the other diets out there? Tried everything else? Well, look no further because we have the REAL answer!" How can *every* program purport to have the real answer? Not to mention, if a real answer truly existed, wouldn't we all be following it by now? If you could personify the diet industry over the last four decades or so, he might ramble on something like this:

> "If you want to lose weight, you need to stop eating all that fat. Because fat makes you fat. Every idiot knows that. So don't eat any fat. Ever. For any reason. Trust me! Follow this plan, and you'll do just fine."
>
> "Okay, *some* fat isn't bad. In fact, I think some is actually good for you. So just eat these fats. But in moderation, of course. Everything in moderation! Do this and you'll definitely lose weight *and* lower your cholesterol. Really."
>
> "Actually, in the absence of carbohydrates, fat doesn't seem to make you fat at all. In fact, a high fat, low carb diet makes you lose fat and lower your cholesterol. I've really got it nailed this time. Do this and you simply can't go wrong."
>
> "Have you tried just drinking protein shakes? A lot of recent research has shown this is foolproof. Really: you can actually lose a *lot* of weight just by drinking protein shakes. Honest. Do it! *Right now, dammit!*"
>
> "Why are you drinking protein shakes! Are you nuts? That's the *worst* thing you can do to your body. Sheesh! Don't you stupid people know anything about basic nutrition? Go back to eating good foods in moderation and you can't go wrong."
>
> "Okay, so now it looks like no matter how you lose weight, eventually the same number of people reach the same goals in about the same amount of time. Further, the maintenance rates are about equal among all diets. So just go back to the moderation thing. Really. I'm positive it will work this time."

"You're not eating in moderation, are you? Maybe you need an appetite suppressant or some of this special herbal tea. You know if you take this Lipotastic Pill, you can eat whatever the hell you want, and the pounds will just melt off. See? Just look at this supermodel climbing out of the pool wearing a bikini. She looked *just like you* last week. Seriously, this is it: do this and you'll lose weight. I'm positive about this now."

"Wait a minute. Are those trans-fats you're eating? What's the matter with you! Those are *evil*. You might as well bake cookies with arsenic. Cut out *all trans-fats immediately* or you'll be dead in seventy-two hours. We're serious this time! Oh, and cut back on fat and carbs while you're at it. Don't you people know anything?"

What's an ordinary consumer to do? I'd say grab a can of Pringles and drown out the noise. That's what I'd do. "Mixed messages?" That has to be the understatement of the century.

Chapter 9

Time to Do Something

I used to scoff at the thought of walking as a mode of exercise. *Exercising*, as every rational person knows, means lifting weights, or running long distances, or doing something that otherwise actually forces you to contract muscle tissue. Walking is what you do to get from your front door to your car. Walking is not exercise.

My thoughts on this were abruptly changed one spring afternoon when The Snouts decided to walk to get lunch instead of taking the car. *Walk!* Can you believe that? Here in America, of all places! It was about one mile each way, and while I did survive the arduous trek, it pretty much knocked me out. I was quite winded and tired by the time we returned. I didn't think swinging my arms and legs back and forth for forty minutes—even just a little—could wear me out like that.

Stunned by hitting 239 pounds on page 50, I began giving some serious thought to the next stage in my life. Not only did I need to lose weight but I was also growing a bit tired of my current occupation. (That's putting it mildly.) I began to have thoughts about a severe career change. Wild fantasies of quitting my job and spending my days working at home as a full time writer began to enter my head. Never mind that I'd never before actually written anything, but I wasn't about to let a couple of things like *no experience* and *no income* stop me. It's also worth noting that I believed this at-home fantasy job of mine would also give me copious amounts of time to exercise and get in shape.

As it turned out, I didn't quit my job and I didn't begin writing for a couple more years. But I did finally get serious about exercising. Weighing nearly two hundred and forty pounds was unacceptable. I thought I'd make at least one part of my fantasy come true by buying Elle Macpherson. (Er, sorry...wrong fantasy.) I mean, I decided to make part of my *work-at-home* fantasy come true by buying a piece of home exercise equipment: a walking machine.

It wasn't a treadmill. It was one of those swingy back and forth walker devices, somewhat akin to Tony Little's *Gazelle* machine. It would work both your arms and legs at the same time. It had a small computing device that counted time elapsed and strides taken and (somehow) could tell you how many calories you burned.*

I tried it out for a while. If you want my own personal, late-night infomercial-like testimonial, here you go: *it was boring as hell.* I thought walking was bad enough. Walking without the benefit of changing scenery is pure torture. To help liven it up a bit, I thought perhaps putting it in front of the television would help. It didn't. It turned television into pure torture. TV was designed for mindless sitting. Let's keep it that way.

The first three months of 1997 did not go well. I tried both dieting and exercising—sometimes at the same time—but just

---

* I never quite understood how it did that It certainly didn't know how tall I was or how much I weighed. Apparently, ten minutes of walking burns the exact same amount of calories for a 240-pound man as it does for a 120-pound woman.

the usual fits and starts. Despite the panic of hitting an all-time high weight and my strongest-ever desire to get back to "normal," I simply could not get it into gear. In April, all that changed. I started walking.

Yes. Walking. I recalled the lunchtime treks that wore me out so easily. And although I got nothing out of the walking machine, I knew that this probably wasn't a bad option at this point. I also had two important things going for me: 1) there were places at work to walk and; 2) there were locker rooms with showers too. I simply had to take advantage of this most excellent arrangement.

I started simple, first by taking short walks between buildings and then by venturing outside. Inside, one could walk for what seemed like a half mile through hallways and walkways connecting the various buildings. Outside, there were miles of trails going in different directions. I had the choice of walking through trees, or open fields, or housing subdivisions. Looking back, it was truly an ideal situation. I wish I had something like that now.

In about twelve weeks, I'd dropped twenty pounds. About six weeks after that, I'd lost another ten. Check out 1997!

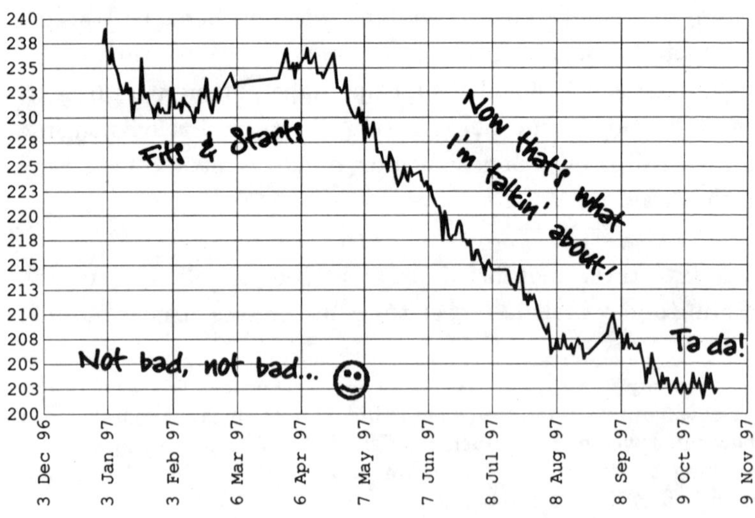

With very few exceptions, I walked five days every week. Each day I walked between forty-five minutes and an hour. Diet-wise, I wasn't following any specific plan, although I tried to watch what I was eating in general. But I'm positive the food had little to do with it. It was all about getting off my butt and *moving*. And do you want to know what the most important thing was? It wasn't boring—not in the least bit. If it were, I can tell you there's *no way* I would have kept at it as long as I did. I really hit my stride, both figuratively and literally. Walking—that activity I'd for so long dismissed as pointless—was absolute bliss. It gave me time to think. Heck, it just gave me time to *breathe*. It was exactly what I needed exactly when I needed it.

And he lived happily ever after.

Hang on, hang on! Not so fast. First, take a look at the next two months:

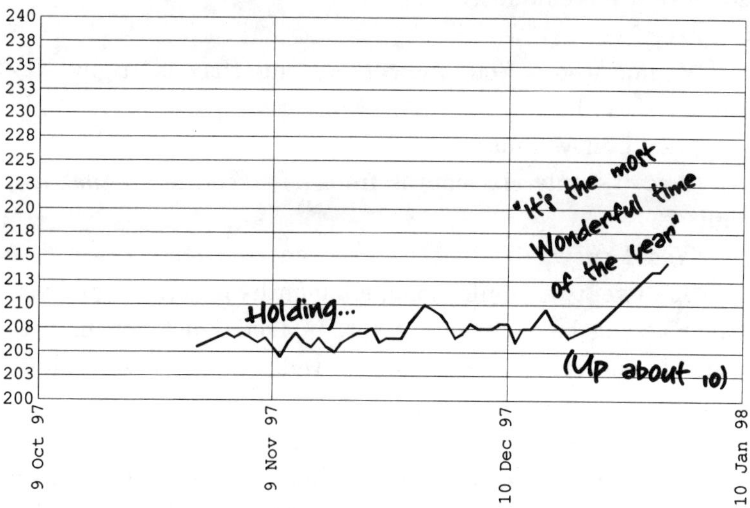

No surprise there, of course. That's just the normal, expected, end-of-year gain. There are no exceptions, even on the best of years. (You know the Third Law.) What's a guy to do?

I could have quit. I could have just given up and let that graph continue on its merry way skyward. Lord knows I've felt like that before (and I'll certainly feel that way again). But not this time. For whatever reason, whatever got my feet moving in April of 1997 kept me going strong in 1998.

I resumed walking. It was still winter, so I stuck to the indoor routes at work. Spring came and I moved outside. I was slowly but surely edging my way back down to the pre-holiday point. Then something interesting happened.

One day in April, my sister Beth phoned. We went through the normal catch-up conversations. She then told me that she finally decided to get on her own health kick. I congratulated her on her decision and wished her luck. That's when she dropped the bomb.

"I'm going to do the Chicago Marathon in October."

I replied with a moment of stunned silence.

"Yeah, that's what most people say," she added.

"A marathon? You want to do a marathon?" I inquired, somewhat incredulously.

"Yes."

"A marathon. You know how long that is, right? It's twenty-six miles."

"Yes. I know," she said.

"And it's only six months from now. You know that too, right?"

"Yes. I know."

"It's twenty-six miles long, six months from now, and you haven't even begun training yet. In fact, I bet you haven't walked more than a mile since—well, probably since high school."

"Yes. I know."

I sat for a moment, thinking about how crazy this all sounded. What was she thinking? How could she just decide to up and do something like this? Marathons take years of training, don't they?

But as I contemplated this whacky plan for a moment, it actually didn't sound like such a bad idea after all. I could see her point. It was a goal. It was something to shoot for. I've always believed *if not for the last minute, nothing would ever get done.* This was a "last minute" if there ever was one. It meant getting into gear.

Then, in the deep recesses of my dusty brain, a tiny ember began to flare. I thought to myself, "*Self, you know something like this could work for you too.*"

Then, much to my own wonder, I said, "I'll do it with you."

"Really?" She asked hopefully.

"Really," I confirmed.

"You know this is twenty-six miles, only six months from now, and you've barely walked more than four miles at once."

She wanted to make sure I hadn't lost my senses.

"Yes. I know."

And so it was on: The Great Marathon Training of 1998. We both decided to keep doing what we were doing, with one sanity check. In June, there was a 20K run in Des Moines called "Dam to Dam." Twenty kilometers works out to roughly half a marathon so this would be a good litmus test of our progress. If we could pull that off in two months, maybe we had a good shot at doubling the distance in just four more months. (That or we had good shot at killing ourselves.)

I was still primarily confined to walking during my lunch hours. For this reason, I couldn't do more than three or four miles a day. But I figured consistency was better than nothing, and I did try to quicken my pace with each passing week.

We were still both *walking*, however. Dam to Dam is clearly a *running* race. We didn't know if we'd be able to walk without getting in the way of the real athletes. I already knew that in these anyone-can-enter races, some people end up walking at least part of the course. So I figured if some people could walk part of it, would anyone notice if a couple people walked all of it. Besides, what's the worst that could happen? We could get turned away and be out thirty bucks. The silver lining in that cloud is we'd be able to watch the race results over beer at a sports bar. Worse things have happened.

The day of the race dawned bright and clear. It looked to be a fine day for road walking (or beer drinking). We took the runner's shuttle up to Saylorville Dam, where the race began. One good thing about this particular race: it runs downstream from the dam to the city. So (most of) the course is downhill. There was one reportedly tough uphill area, but this year's course went around it, due to construction. (Yay!)

Beth and I looked around. The view was beautiful. Facing the starting line, Saylorville Lake stretched for miles to our left. To our right, about eleven miles away, we could see the city skyline, a gray mass shimmering on the edge of sight in the early morning sun. We looked at each other and pointed. "We're *walking* there!" It was hard for me to believe the day had finally arrived and we were actually here. We were really going to do this.

In order to minimize our impact on the rest of the racers, we decided to begin about forty-five minutes before the official start of the race. My idea was to put at least three miles between the frontrunners and us. We pulled our shoelaces tight, moseyed toward the start line, and with no fanfare or even as much as a starting gun, we began the "race."

One thing about walking: it's not much to look at. It's nothing anyone would call exciting, and that was probably our best cover. "Don't mind us! We're just a couple of runners checking out the course!"

A short way past the end of the dam, we hit our first check. It wasn't entirely obvious which way we had to go. The typical runner gives no thought to this. The typical runner simply follows the pack. We looked around then approached a police officer standing at a barricade. We asked him which way the course went. "Um..." he hesitated for a moment, glancing from side to side. "That way." He pointed towards our right. So off to the right we went, beginning to wonder if the sports bar wouldn't have been the best option after all. We did, of course, feel a bit funny just meandering down the road all by ourselves. A couple people remarked to us in a good-natured fashion, "Getting a little head start, are we?" We just waved—and agreed. That's exactly what we were doing.

I had hoped to take between twelve and fifteen minutes for each mile. I'd been able to finish one or two miles in the past under twelve minutes, but I found it exceedingly difficult. Walking any faster than that meant running. (And I simply cannot run.) Anything over fifteen minutes per mile would be unacceptably slow. So you can imagine my dismay when twenty minutes went by and we still hadn't seen a mile marker.

"We can't be going *that* slow," I said to Beth.

"Maybe the first mile isn't marked?" she offered.

"Why would they not mark the first mile?" I mumbled to myself. It didn't make sense.

Only a few more minutes passed when we saw the first mile marker. This may have been my first-ever road race, but I was pretty darn sure that they would use "1" to represent the first mile marker and not a "2." But there it was right in front of us: "2." I pondered this curiosity for a moment.

"We took the wrong turn," I said, solving the riddle.

"Huh?" Beth asked.

"Back there. The policeman. He pointed us in the wrong direction."

"Oh well. Nothing we can do about it now," she stated.

"Nope. I'm just thoroughly pleased we're not walking twenty-two minute miles."

We walked together for another couple of miles. It wasn't long before the frontrunners passed us. We stepped clear out of the way, and let the bulk of the crowd move by, unhindered by a couple of oddballs who decided to walk a running race. Some way after that, curious about my own capabilities, I asked her if it would be all right if we split up.

"I just need to know how fast I can comfortably go. I know it's faster than this."

"That's fine! I'll see you at the finish!" she replied and sent me off with a wave.

I was a bit torn, however. We were having an enjoyable walk. After all, how often do you get to do something like this? Still, I had to know what it was like. I needed to test myself now if I had any chance of doing an entire marathon in four months. Besides, we would be walking the Big One together in October. We would have plenty of time to walk and talk then.

To make a twenty-kilometer story short, I finished the race. In fact, I even finished *running*, if you can believe it. For some reason, walking through the chute at the end didn't feel like proper race etiquette.

The race was a thoroughly enjoyable experience too. *Officially,* I finished in two hours and twelve minutes: a mile pace of ten minutes and thirty-seven seconds. Of course, considering that we started *well* before the gun *and* took a nice short cut at the very beginning, it probably took me more like three hours to do maybe eleven and a half miles. The time didn't matter much to me. What I found most important is that I did it, and *it wasn't a big deal.* It didn't matter that I'd only walked four miles before. I had got myself into shape. True, I still hadn't lost as much weight as I'd wanted (or even expected, given the workout levels). But I learned I could handle it—and that was saying a lot.

I hung out by the finish line for about a half hour when Beth came down the chute. We both felt pretty darn good about our accomplishments to date. When the weekend was over, she returned to Chicago. I returned to my workouts.

Chapter 10

How to Go on a Diet

It just dawned on me I've done a lot of talking about dieting, but really haven't explained how to go about doing one yourself. So, for the twelve of you reading this book who've never been on a diet, I thought I'd run you through the complete process. The rest of you—the pros—can safely skip to page 100 and read all about nutrition. You're welcome to stay and check my work, of course, but I'm sure I have this particular topic nailed.

Step 1: Flip the Switch

The first step, of course, is to make The Decision. The Decision usually isn't a conscious one, which is the main problem. It operates on a subconscious (if not completely unconscious) level. It's controlled by what I like to call The Switch.

The Switch is either on or it's off. There is no dimmer setting. You can't be "kinda on." When it's on, you can stick to your diet no matter what. When it's off, nothing—and I mean *nothing*—can keep you on the diet. So you see the only trick to losing weight is getting control of The Switch.

The problem is, as I've stated, you have no control over

The Switch. Sorry. That's just the way we're wired. The only way to get it turned on is by experiencing some earth-shattering event. It's the sudden realization of *Oh my God, I'm huger than I've ever been and I just can't take this any more.* Once this happens, you're actually more than halfway there. The trigger can be any one of the following:

- Can't tie your own shoes any more.
- Suddenly have to buy size 16 pants.
- Just one seat won't cut it on the airplane.
- Terribly winded after one flight of stairs.
- Playing with kids induces heart failure.
- That photo. That awful, awful photo.
- Elle Macpherson turns you down again.
- Can't get up without making that grunting noise.
- Did I mention that awful photo?

Step 2: Pick a Program

The second step is to choose your weapon. As discussed earlier in the book, there are hundreds of weight loss tools at your disposal. Which one you pick doesn't matter much since The Switch is now on. Just find something that doesn't make you sick to your stomach or turn you into a raving lunatic and you'll do just fine.

Step 3: Plan Your Meals

It's funny, no matter which diet you pick you pretty much end up with the same basic approach. The idea is to stop doing whatever you've been doing and start eating the "right" way. You'll be introduced to terms like "portion control" and "moderation". You'll get all excited and make that very first grocery trip where you enthusiastically buy all the good foods and wistfully pass up all the stuff you like.

The good news is you don't have to come up with the meal plans yourself. These are provided for you by your best-selling diet book's famous author person. The meals are broken out into carefully measured portions, and are to be consumed at carefully scheduled times of the day. On the surface, it looks like normal food. But as you get into it, you'll find there's nothing natural about eating this way at all. If The Switch is on, that's okay: you'll stick to it come hell or high water. If the switch is off, however, you'll probably do what ninety percent of us do. It goes something like this.

Day 1	
Breakfast	One slice of reduced-calorie, sugar-free bread, toasted. One teaspoon of fat-free, butter-like spread. Three ounces of fresh melon. Eight ounces of skim milk.
Lunch	One half cup of tuna salad made with fat-free mayonnaise. Two slices of low-calorie, sugar-free bread. One slice each of lettuce and tomato. One cup of water.
Snack	One quarter cup of fat-free cottage cheese. One cup of water.
Dinner	Three ounces of skinned, grilled chicken breast, lightly salted. Salad with mixed greens, cucumbers, fat-free croutons and fat-free dressing. One cup of fresh strawberries for dessert.

Day 2	
Breakfast	One cup of cooked oatmeal. Eight ounces of skim milk. A cup of coffee—the "no caffeine" rule was stupid. Caffeine doesn't make you fat.
Lunch	Avocado and mixed greens salad. One package of fat-free soda crackers. A diet coke.

Snack	Rice cake with one teaspoon peanut butter. One cup of water.
Dinner	Poached salmon with black beans and rice. One wholegrain cracker. One cup of fresh strawberries for dessert. Eight ounces of skim milk.

Day 3	
Breakfast	A bowl of Rice Krispies with milk. One banana. Two pieces of toast with actual margarine. Orange juice. Coffee with half-and-half.
Lunch	Lunch meeting at work, deli ordered in: One turkey club sandwich. Dill pickle spear. One package of Lays potato chips. One chocolate chip cookie. One can of Coca-Cola.
Snack	One "fun size" *3 Musketeers* bar. (It's okay, because they're lighter than air.)
Dinner	Spaghetti and meatballs. Garlic bread. Salad with thousand island dressing. Ice cream.

Day 4	
Breakfast	Starbucks Banana Coconut Frappuccino on the way into work. One Krispy Kreme donut at work, thanks to Chet in accounting.
Lunch	Six-inch Subway Sweet Onion Chicken Teriyaki sandwich. One bag of Cool Ranch Doritos. One sixteen ounce Dr. Pepper.

Snack	One leftover Krispy Kreme donut. Another Dr. Pepper.
Dinner	Kids have soccer practice at 5:30, so you run by the McDonald's drive-thru: Quarter Pounder with Cheese. Large fries. Large Coke.

Day 5	
Breakfast	Nothing.
Lunch	Nothing. You're really trying to make up for the last day or two.
Snack	One bag of chips out of the vending machine. Oh, man, you *almost* made it.
Dinner	Day 5 is, of course, Friday, which is, as everyone knows, pizza night: Six slices of deep-dish pepperoni and Italian sausage pizza. Three bottles of beer.
Snack	One bag of "movie butter" microwave popcorn during family DVD night. One or two more beers. Chips and dip.

If, on the other hand, you're in the minority of dieters with The Switch on, this won't happen to you. (Yet.) For now, you'll follow the prescribed plan religiously, and do quite well.

Step 4: Exercise

Only twelve percent* of all dieters actually embark on an accompanying exercise program. If you're one of the few who do, congratulations. You have my respect. If on the other hand, you're with us in the majority, then you're probably wonder-

* Or maybe it's twenty-seven percent. I'm not sure. I made up the number a long time ago.

ing what a common exercise program looks like. Fortunately, you've come to the right place because that's exactly what I'm going to show you. Let's start by looking at the different ways to exercise:

- Walking (burns 500 calories an hour)
- Aerobics (800 calories an hour)
- Running (900 calories an hour)
- Stair machine (1000 calories an hour)
- Dusting the exercise equipment (90 calories a month)
- Writing a check to the gym (20 calories a month)
- Channel surfing (10 calories a day)
- Twelve ounce curls (negative 180 calories an hour)

This is just a tiny sampling of the possible activities. Even the softest of couch potatoes would have trouble not finding something to do. Now let's look at how a few activities actually work on a daily basis:

Exercise	Common Regimen
Pilates	1. Join an exercise club or buy a DVD. 2. Get up Monday morning; do the routine for one hour. 3. Get up late Tuesday morning: do the routine for forty minutes. 4. Sleep in on Wednesday. You deserve it. 5. Get up on time Thursday, but watch TV instead. 6. Forget Friday... 7. ...and the weekend. 8. Next Monday, repeat.
Bowflex	1. Purchase $1,100 unit. 2. Eagerly set it up on Saturday. 3. Try it out on Monday. 4. Convert to a clothes hanger on Tuesday.

Racquetball	1. Join a gym. 2. Find a partner. 3. Play once. 4. Burn further calories by playing the game called "schedule conflict."
Tai Chi	1. Find Martial Arts studio offering classes. 2. Enjoy it for a couple days. 3. Ultimately, get your Chen mixed up with your Yang, and leave in disgrace.

It doesn't take much imagination to see where the rest of this is going. Except for the chosen few, sticking with a regular exercise program is darn near impossible.

Step 5: Maintenance

About two percent* of all dieters reach their goal and enter what's commonly known as the maintenance phase. The idea is just that: maintain your new weight. At least that's the concept. Unfortunately, the majority of dieters use the maintenance phase to gain back all the weight they lost. (In case you needed any more evidence to support the "diets don't work" hypothesis.)

Most experts agree with me too. They will tell you that the key to successful, long-term weight loss isn't about dieting at all, but instead a "lifestyle change." In short, it means you can't hop off a diet, return to your old eating habits, and expect to keep the weight off. (Yet another helpful tip from The Obvious Files.)

But here's the trick. The lifestyle change is a wee bit easier said than done. Just forget everything you've been doing for the past several decades and do something else instead. If you can do that, you can not only lose the weight but also keep it off for good.

---

* Did you know that fifty-seven percent of all statistics are made up on the fly?

It's a very popular concept because it simultaneously sounds both very wise and so forehead-slapping obvious. "Of course! I must change my lifestyle! Why didn't I think of that?" Are you overweight, have a crappy job, medical bills piling up, and the utility companies cutting you off? Just change your lifestyle, silly!

So it's a sad fact that changing your lifestyle somewhat hinges on having actual control over your *current* lifestyle. But if you can swing it, I definitely recommend it. Some common strategies for permanent lifestyle change involve:

- Never eating out again.
- Replacing your pantry door with a brick wall.
- Selling your refrigerator.
- Serving meals in matchboxes.
- Sleeping twenty-two hours a day.

These are all relatively minor adjustments, so you should have no problems whatsoever maintaining your new, low weight.

Step 6: Falling off the Wagon

Once you've completed the maintenance phase, you're ready to completely fall off the wagon. If you were on a low fat diet, this means heading down to the local bar and grill, ordering up *The Chubbyman Platter* and eating until the grease seeps from your pores. If you were on a Detox diet, you head to Wendy's. If you were doing low carb, you hit the Pizza Hut buffet and pile your plate with the thickest pan pizza offered.

But you tell yourself this is okay. You've been good. You deserve it. Besides, what's the worst that could happen? Unfortunately, the very next morning the low fat dieter whips up bacon and eggs while the low carb guy fixes hash browns. No problem, though. It's just breakfast. You'll definitely do better by dinner—tomorrow night. Or Tuesday. Or maybe January.

Yeah, that'll work. You'll be ready in January.

Step 7: Re-dieting

Guess what? It's January—time to start up your diet again! The hope and promise of a new year is your greatest weapon. Your fat cells don't stand a chance. Most people will hop right back on the diet they had the most success with. A few others may try something different. Me, I just recommend that you go to Amazon.com, see what the #1 best-seller is and follow that. It *has* to work, right? Otherwise, why would so many people be buying that book?

With your new (or old) diet in hand, make that optimistic trip to the grocery store and stock up on whatever it is this particular diet requires.

Follow the plan to the letter, just as you did before, only this time *do it forever*. It's a foolproof plan.

Chapter 11

A Beginner's Guide to Nutrition

A wide variety of nutrients keeps the human body functioning properly. Things like vitamins and minerals are collectively known as *micronutrients.* I have to be honest; I really don't know much about these guys. I can't tell you much more about them other than the fact that they are naturally shaped like Flintstones characters. Therefore, in this chapter, I'm going to tackle the big three foods or *macronutrients.* They are carbohydrates, proteins, and fats. Let's go through them one at a time.

Food #1: Carbohydrates

Ah, the naughty carbohydrate. We've sure heard a *lot* about you over the years. You make us fat. You make us insane. We must never associate with the likes of *you* again. In fact, I've even heard there are some whacky people out there with the crazy notion that the body actually *needs* carbohydrates to function. Ha! Who could ever think that?

What? You mean to say that's actually true? Carbohydrates *aren't* bad? So what's with all this noise about carbs if the innocent carbohydrate molecule is necessary to live?

It's easily explained. The individual carbohydrate isn't to blame. It's our penchant for consuming seventy five times the necessary amount. *That's* the real problem.

Carbohydrates are made out of carbon, hydrogen, and oxygen atoms. They generally follow a basic CH_2O molecular pattern. (Looks like carbon and water, doesn't it? Hence the name: carbohydrate.) Let's examine the different flavors.

Monosaccharides. These are the simplest carbohydrates in our diets. They are small sugar molecules and when ingested require no processing whatsoever as this is our body's primary fuel in its purest form. The three monosaccharides are glucose (typically known as *dextrose* in the food industry), galactose, and fructose. Yum.

Disaccharides. Take two monosaccharide molecules, glue them together, toss out one water molecule and you have one of these. They stand at the next rung up the complexity ladder. Disaccharides include sucrose, lactose, and maltose. Sucrose is simple table sugar and is formed by combining glucose and fructose. A cookie just isn't a cookie without sucrose, that's for sure.

Polysaccharides. Now we're in the realm of complex carbohydrates. This polymer of many monosaccharides manifests itself in our diets primarily as starch. Typical sources are potatoes, rice, grains, beans, and the like. Due to their complexity, they are not absorbed in the body as quickly as simple sugars. It takes more work to break them down into glucose. Ironically enough, when your body ends up with excess glucose, it reassembles it into a polysaccharide called glycogen, for short-term energy storage. It's like you can make your own potatoes. (Which explains your thighs.)

Fiber. This is a non-starch polysaccharide. It is indigestible and primarily just passes right through you—but that's its very strength. It helps to maintain the health of your entire digestive tract and can help lower cholesterol. Odds are you're not getting enough of it. So you'd better get working on that, okay?

This is, of course, just the short list. There are others, as you might expect. The complete study of biochemistry is left as an exercise to the reader. It's a fascinating field. In fact, I myself am planning to study it more just as soon as I finish this donut.

So, now that you're a carbohydrate expert, how do you go about making the right food choices? Good carbs, bad carbs, whole grains, fruits, fiber, Count Chocula Cereal—it can all be so overwhelming. And the food industry, always catering to our perceptions, is no help. Take, for example, bread. At the point when whole grains started gaining popularity, the industry leapt into action by putting the word WHEAT on bread packaging. Of course, bread was *always* made of wheat. But using big letters made a connection in the heads of those who had "whole wheat" on the brain. As soon as the consumer caught on, they then added brown food coloring to the bread to make it look wheatier. "If it's brown, it must be good!" thought the consumer. Well, no. It's still made from highly refined white flour. It just looks brown.

The bottom line is you have to be on your guard. There are plenty of places to look for information. The good news is that the basics don't change. That is, if whole grain wheat is good for you this year, it will probably be good for you next year too. (Unless someone comes along with an article called, *The Truth about Whole Grain Wheat.*) Anyway, enough about sugars. Let's move on to our second macronutrient, protien. Or possibly even protein.*

---

* I never can spell it right. Sometimes I think the "i before e" rule is made up of nothing *but* exceptions. Beige? Neither? Weird? Heist? Veil? Does that look like an "i before e, except after c" rule to you?

Food #2: Proteins

When you hear the term "protein" in a dietary context, it's very likely you immediately think of foods such as meat, eggs, or nuts. We use the word almost daily, but very few of us really know exactly what they are or why we need them.

While carbohydrates provide fuel to your body's trillions of little subsystems, proteins essentially *are* the subsystems. Proteins provide structural integrity to cells. They're a major source of nitrogen—a critical element conspicuously absent from carbs and fats. Some proteins are quite active, parading about your body as enzymes or hormones or even neurotransmitters. They help your red blood cells get oxygen around your system. Proteins are definitely the workaholics of your organic self.

Now, with that knowledge, guess how much protein your body needs on a daily basis to keep functioning. Ten grams? Fifty? Two hundred? BZZZT! Oh, I'm sorry, that was the wrong answer. The answer we were looking for was *zero.* That's right; your body requires absolutely no protein whatsoever. What it *does* require, however, is amino acids, and that's where the protein comes in. Remember high school science? Amino acids are the building blocks of protein.

Your body has two ways of getting the amino acids it requires: some of them it can synthesize on its own out of other nutrients; the others (known collectively as "essential amino acids") must be taken from consumed proteins.*

The names of amino acids sound like alien races you might find in a Star Trek episode: Leucine, Methionine, or Lysine. One or two have even found their way into everyday language. Have you ever eaten a big Thanksgiving meal and then got *really sleepy* afterwards? Somehow back in the 1990s or so, tryptophan was identified as the culprit. This amino

---

* It's interesting that the body consumes proteins just to break them down into amino acids; only to *then* turn around and recombine them into the proteins your body actually needs.

acid is present in turkey meat and it does indeed have a documented narcotic affect. However, it only works in a pure form and with no other proteins present. (Never mind that it's also found in chicken, beef, beans, and other protein-rich foods, but they're never blamed for inexplicable fits of drowsiness.) Given that, it's hardly the cause of you falling asleep during the football game every fourth Thursday of each November. If that's the case, then why *do* you feel sleepy after a big turkey-day dinner? Gee, I wonder. You think maybe it's the 7,000-calorie meal you just gobbled down? Every ounce of energy in your body has been sent to process the caloric onslaught. There's not much energy left for anything else.

So how much protein does your body need? The answer is, in exact scientific terms, "just enough." Too little, and your body will start breaking down its own tissues to get the amino acids it requires. Too much, and you can overtax key systems, such as your liver and kidneys. Experts and laypersons alike disagree on the exact details. A general rule of thumb is a 1:1000 protein-to-weight ratio, meaning, "one gram of protein per day per kilogram of body weight." That works out to about ninety grams a day for a two hundred pound couch potato.

So that's pretty much protein for you! Sorry it's not very exciting or controversial. Yep, your body needs it. Yep, you better eat some. Yawn. Anyway, we're all getting anxious to talk about our most favorite food of all! Wait no longer, 'cuz here it comes!

Food #3: Fats

With the many diets and weight loss programs we've all seen, tried, or otherwise experienced over the last few decades, no one message stands out quite as much as *fat is bad*. Oh, I'm sure it began innocently enough. Simple math initially told us that fat wasn't a good idea. It has more calories per gram than either carbohydrates or proteins. Therefore, eating one kilogram of Crisco will deliver far more calories to your body than the equivalent in cotton candy. But as we began to look beyond the simple issues of excess energy, we saw other concerns. The fat you eat clogs your arteries. It can lead to heart disease. It can kill your liver. It causes cancer. It's probably the reason Susie went and left you for some foreign guy.

It's important to note that eating fat in and of itself does not make you fat. That is, you don't eat a cheeseburger and suddenly a cheeseburger pops up in your thigh. It's not even as simple as the fat extracted from the cheeseburger goes straight to your thighs. Remember, your body is a machine and food is its fuel. Everything you eat is broken down into basic components and taken to one of three places:

1. Usable fuel is carted around the body and burned.
2. Excess fuel is hauled off for storage.
3. Everything else ends up at your city's waste treatment facility.

Fat is actually good. We tend to forget that little tidbit. Fat benefits the body in many ways. It helps build tissues. (It is, after all, what your cell walls are made of.) It helps with the absorption of vitamins and other nutrients. It helps keep you warm. Fat is good. Don't be so mean to it.

So why the bad rap, if fat itself isn't bad? Well, you already know the answer to that question.* In short, the truth about fat can be summed up in two parts: 1) the word "fat" is used to describe not one thing, but a wide variety of compounds; and 2) there's a difference between an avocado and a family size bag of Funyuns. In other words, we need to find the proper fats and eat them in the correct quantities. Fat only has this bad reputation because we eat such large volumes of it (and we tend to carry the excess to the beach as we mingle with our fellow whales).

---

* I bet you read that "Truth about Fat" article didn't you?

The large number of different fat molecules combined with the fact that we generally use one word for all of them naturally leads to confusion. Don't feel bad if you can't make heads or tails of it all. It's possible to make sense of it without needing to know that fatty acids are just chains of specifically-arranged hydrogen and carbon and oxygen atoms or the fact that when a carbon atom decides to bond with only one hydrogen atom plus double bond with another carbon atom, we call that a monounsaturated fatty acid. Instead, popular culture just likes to talk about fats being either *good* or *bad*.

Good fats are the ones found in hamburgers, French fries, movie popcorn butter, cheese omelets, and Chicago deep-dish pizzas. Bad fats are the ones found in fish. Oh, wait a minute. I'm mixing up *good* with *good tasting*. Odd how that works.

So I guess we have our rule. If it tastes really, really good, then it's bad for you. Therefore, never eat anything that tastes good or you will have a heart attack. All kidding aside, I think knowing the breakdown of the different types of fats *is* important, so here goes. (Who says a humor book can't be edumacational too.)

Monounsaturated. These fats primarily come from plants. They are liquid at room temperature, and for that reason commonly go by the word "oil." You find them in peanuts, cashews, avocados, and olives. They can reduce bad cholesterol in your bloodstream while raising the good. These fats get a universal stamp of approval.

Polyunsaturated. You find these fats in plants and seafood. Like monos, they too are liquid at room temperature. Common sources include soy, sesame, corn, and sunflower oils. These fats reduce bad cholesterol more than monounsaturated fats, but do not affect levels of good cholesterol. Soy oil is the reason mayonnaise, in moderation, isn't so bad for you after all.

Saturated. These fats are usually associated with animal products: beef, poultry, pork, milk, and cheese, to name a few. As a rule of thumb, saturated fats are solid at room temperature. Some plants have saturated fats, such as coconuts and pistachios, but it's not as common. I also hate to break it to you, but cocoa butter falls in this category. So watch the chocolate. They have the worst impact on cholesterol in your bloodstream, but are not completely without merit. They can help the immune system and even contribute to bone building.

Hydrogenated. These fats are primarily a product of the food industry. They start as unsaturated fats, but have hydrogen gas bubbled through them causing them to change from unsaturated to saturated. This is how something benign like vegetable oil can turn into margarine. Hydrogenated fats are closely linked to heart disease. The only real benefit they provide to humanity is that they make the best cookies.

Trans Fats. These fats are rare in the natural world. They are created through the hydrogenation process. Although chemically they are unsaturated, they share none of the goodness listed above. They are not required by the body and are to blame for many health woes. While people have preached against them for decades, it's only recently that "trans fat free" has become a marketing tool.

Maybe that's more than you ever wanted to know about fat. Or maybe not. There's no shortage of books on the subject if you want to learn more about this fascinating topic. I tell you, there's nothing quite like spending a rainy day in bed, with a tall glass of whole milk and a big plate of sugar cookies, and reading Dr. Avery P. Rutherman's latest book, *Plasminogen Activator Inhibitor-1 and its Relation to Adipose Tissues*.

Fat Free!

Have you ever played that party game where a few sentences are passed by whisper from person to person until the last person in the room recites them out loud? Invariably the output of this game bears little resemblance to the input. I have a feeling this is not unlike what happened with the low-fat phenomenon that raged unchecked for decades. People began to honestly (yet incorrectly) repeat everything they'd heard about how bad fat was. By the time it reached the other side of the room, the original message was unrecognizable. But that didn't matter, because the People Had Spoken. They now knew that the only key to losing weight was by cutting fat and they set out to find foods with as little fat as possible. The food industry, ever eyeing the next dollar, obliged us by providing every sort of low-fat, fat-free, and cholesterol-free product imaginable.

The overall result, as we know, was not good. Many, many factors contributed to the failure of the low fat diet. For now, I'd like to focus on one that I haven't seen discussed much.

They say imitation is the sincerest form of flattery. In some cases, I suppose that can be true. But at other times, it can be just plain weird. I believe the latter is the way it is with food. As we now know, you can't really lose weight until the Switch in your head has been flipped and you can't really keep the Switch flipped unless you make the fundamental lifestyle change. This is where things get a little strange.

The operative word in "fundamental lifestyle change" is *change.* Yet change is the very thing we seem to be completely incapable of doing. Think about it. When we collectively made the decision to switch to low-fat diets, what did we do? Did we eat more carrots, spinach and lean skinless chicken breasts? Sure, a few of us did—at least for a while. But the overwhelming majority of us started looking for low fat versions of the crap we'd been stuffing ourselves with for years. Don't fix a pot of vegetable soup. Grab a box of fat-free cookies instead. Why bother preparing a fruit salad? It's so much easier to dig into a bag of Olestra potato chips. Your dramatic lifestyle "change" is anything *but* that. All you've done is swapped ingredients. You haven't changed your behavior. You haven't changed your caloric intake. You haven't started burning more calories. Before and After snapshots of your cupboard would probably be indistinguishable to the naked eye. (As would the Before and After snapshots of your body.)

Let's say one of your favorite foods before your diet was a turkey sandwich with lettuce, cheese, and mayonnaise. After you make your major lifestyle change, your favorite is now a turkey sandwich with lettuce, fat-free cheese, and fat-free mayonnaise. Wow. Really big change there, champ. Let's analyze the situation by breaking it down into parts. First up is the cheese.

Fat-free cheese.

Cheese without fat.

Cheese made out of...well, frankly, I have no idea. All I know is that it tastes like plastic. And what's the point? Sure, it has fewer calories and less fat—but at what cost? Let's look at the high-level numbers first. For a one ounce serving:

	Frankencheese	Natural Cheese
Calories	24	68
Fat	0.13 g	5.63 g
Cholesterol	1.78 mg	17.83 mg
Sodium	248 mg	106 mg
Carbs	2.2 g	0.2 g
Protein	3.64 g	4.23 g

There are definitely pros and cons to each. The most striking difference is in the top two stats. The natural cheese has 44 more calories and more than 5 grams of fat. While this figure might make the low-fat crowd cower in fear, is this difference really all that important in the long run? If you're on a 1,800 calorie per day diet, the real cheese is only 2.44% of your total daily intake.

Now let's look at what you're eating. Real cheese is made out of milk and... well, basically just milk and the enzymes that converted the milk into cheese.* Our so-called healthful fat-free alternative cheese is made out of (and I'll quote one popular brand): skim milk, water, milk protein concentrates, whey, dried corn syrup, sodium phosphate, salt, sodium citrate, sorbic acid, carrageenan, cellulose gum, artificial color, milkfat, artificial flavor, sodium tripolyphosphate, citric acid, enzymes, calcium phosphate, natural flavor, vitamin A palmitate, and cheese culture.

Our collective obsession with "fat free or die!" apparently blinds us to all else. Are we really to believe this list of ingredients (many of which aren't even recognized by my spell-checker) is better for us because it saves us a couple dozen calories and a few grams of fat? Is this kind of trade-off really worth it? It's like driving around the parking lot for twenty minutes trying to find a spot close to the door before finally heading into the gym to do your treadmill workout. What's the point? It's a false saving.

And while these strange ingredients might be perfectly harmless in low doses, what happens when they begin to take a steadily larger and larger portion of your diet? Or when they're mixed with other oddball ingredients from some other Franken-product? I can't believe every single possible combination and quantity has been tested.

I'm sure you've read the magazine articles that say, "Just cut out 50 calories a day and you can lose five pounds in a year." They're not lying. Technically speaking, the math pans out. But eating isn't about being technical or rational. You know darn well that if you cut out fifty calories from your

---

* Essentially cheese is nothing more than milk with most its water removed. (Almost nine-tenths of cow's milk is water.) Different cheeses are distinguished by: 1) what kind of milk; 2) how much of the water is removed; and most importantly 3), *how* it's removed. Once the water is gone, all you're left with is fat, protein, sugar, and various minerals.

lunch, you'll be *so* pleased with your amazing display of willpower that you'll have three scoops of ice cream for dessert instead of two. My recommendation is to eat the real cheese and skip the ice cream altogether.

Next on our new and improved sandwich: the fat free mayonnaise. Real mayonnaise *is* fat. It's primarily made from soybean oil and eggs. A one-tablespoon serving size is fourteen grams. Three of those grams are from calorie-free sources (like water), leaving eleven caloric grams. Each serving has eleven grams of fat. You don't have to be a dietician to do the math: one hundred percent of its calories are from fat.

Logic dictates that if regular mayonnaise *is* fat then fat-free mayonnaise *cannot* be mayonnaise at all. So what is it? Well once 98% of the real ingredients have been removed, they add in various starches, sugars, and gums (extraordinarily similar to our above "cheese" product). While you may end up with fewer calories, it's important to remember these new calories are now made up of materials much more readily converted to glucose. With the real stuff, your body will take its time processing it (leaving you feeling satiated for longer). The fake stuff hits the bloodstream quicker, induces false hunger, and helps bring about all those insulin problems we were talking about before. How's that for a lifestyle change?

The term I like to use for this strange syndrome where your new diet gradually takes on the qualities of the diet it was meant to replace is *emulation*. The low-fat dieter does anything to emulate a high-fat diet. ("These fat-free cookies are awesome! I'm going to have *another* box of them!") The low-carb dieter strains to emulate high-carb diets. ("Have you tried the new pancake mix with sugar-free syrup? Set me up with another stack of 'em!") As soon as you see your new diet begin to emulate your old, bad eating habits, you've left the path of wisdom, Grasshopper.

I think the worst offender in this category is the "tastes like the real thing" recipe. We've all seen them. "Here's a fat-free ice cream recipe that tastes like the real thing!" Or "here's a gluten free brownie that tastes like the real thing!" Or, the worst offender of all, "Here are some low-carb 'mashed potatoes' made from cauliflower— it tastes just like the real thing!" I'm sorry, people, but the only thing that *tastes like the real thing* is the real thing itself. If you believe that cauliflower can somehow be prepared to taste like potatoes, then I have some ocean front property in Missouri for sale.

I'm not saying I haven't fallen for this myself. I've consumed a fair number of sugar free candy bars somehow thinking I was sticking to the plan. The theory is that this is supposed to satisfy your craving for the real thing. But I believe it only *increases* your desire for the real thing because the emulated version is never going to stack up.

If you're one of the lucky few who's managed to get the Switch flipped on, then *by all means* take advantage of that. Don't pretend your diet is something it isn't. Don't go over to the dark side. If you're going to make a lifestyle change then *make a change*, for Pete's sake. Actually, forget about Pete. Do it for *your* sake. (Unless, of course, you are Pete.)

Don't pretend. Don't go through the motions. You're only letting yourself down otherwise.

Chapter 12

Now to Keep Doing Something

With the 20K "run" behind me, it was time to focus seriously on the upcoming marathon—a mere one hundred and twenty five days away. On the one hand, I felt like I had all the time in the world. At the beginning of June, the month of October feels years in the future, after all. In all reality, it was right around the corner. Four months is not much time at all, given my growing to-do list:

- Plan summer walking schedule.
- Finalize training diet.
- Buy new shoes.
- Stock up on aspirin.
- Book the ambulance.
- Update last will and testament.
- Notify next of kin.

My walking schedule changed in two ways. First, in order to avoid overloading myself, I cut workweek walking down to just Monday, Wednesday, and Friday. These were fast, three-mile walks, still taken over lunch hours. I was thankful again for the at-work showering facilities. (As were my co-workers.) Second, the stamina-building Saturdays began. These days were carefully designed to ~~break one's spirit~~ get one's body ready for the long haul.

The first of these days was a ten-mile walk. I remember thinking it wouldn't be any problem at all, since it was a full two miles shorter than the Dam to Dam course, and that walk wasn't bad at all.

I was wrong. It was murder.

There is a *huge* difference between a race day and a practice day. A race day is an event, packed with people and full of excitement. Your body is pumped and you're never more ready for anything. On a race day, you can fly to the moon and back. A practice day is lonely and hard. At best they're boring and at worst they're grueling. There is no starting gun. There is no one cheering you on. You are completely on your own. These are the days that truly test an athlete's resolve. (Yes, you read that right. I just called myself an athlete. Pretty funny, huh?)

Worst of all, I'm not a morning person. I live for sleeping in. Hard training on Saturdays meant giving up my favorite day to sleep in. Summer was waxing, so getting an early start was necessary just to keep from overheating. (Although, now that I look back on it, I think my best bet *would* have been to walk at high noon. That would have enabled me to pass out immediately and miss most of the actual walking. But noooo, I just had to do everything by the book, didn't I?)

The walking schedule was provided by Team in Training, commonly known as TNT. I'm not quite sure why they went with "TNT" instead of their real initials, which would have been much better T-shirts if you ask me.

Team in Training was started in 1988. A man named Bruce Cleland decided to do two things: 1) run the New York City Marathon, and 2) raise money for leukemia research. His daughter was a leukemia survivor and the famous running event seemed like the perfect opportunity to raise money and awareness. He assembled a team of thirty-eight runners and together they raised $322,000 for the Westchester/Hudson Valley Chapter of The Leukemia & Lymphoma Society.

Did you catch that number? More than *three hundred thousand dollars*! Let me get my calculator out for a second. That comes out to $8,473.68 per team member. I have two daughters who sell Girl Scout cookies so I *know* what it's like to raise money. Believe me, $8,473.68 is nothing to sneeze at. In the nearly twenty years since, more than $660 million has been raised by hundreds of thousands of volunteers across the country. Wow.

In 1998, Beth was one of those hundreds of thousands. And fortunately, TNT no longer requires participants to raise $8,473.68 apiece. Instead, a mere $1,500 is now required. In return for fundraising efforts, TNT provides training programs, clinics, support, and group sessions—not to mention financial help at the event itself, from hotel accommodations to race entry fees. All that and they *still* manage to make sure 74% of every dollar goes directly to the cause.

Beth raised her $1,500 and then some. My plan all along had been to just tag along with her, more or less. This was, after all, still her big idea. For that reason, I did not sign up for the TNT program. In spite of that, I did go ahead and raise an additional $550 for her on my own. I considered it my tag-along fee.

The official Team in Training plan called for a ten-mile walk on this first of many endurance days. As I already mentioned, it was simply awful. Never mind the fact I had to get up early. Never mind the fact that there were no cheering crowds. If those were my only hurdles, I think I could have managed it without any problems.

But problems I had, right from the start. Obstacles I never anticipated popped up out of nowhere. Let's look at the major ones:

Problem #1: **Ambition**. (Or lack thereof.) I'm sure to the outside observer I looked very strong and dedicated. After all, I had been at this walking thing, non-stop, for a good year already. I had completed a 20K race. I was on track for a full marathon. I never missed a day of practice. Bruce Jenner would have looked up to me—maybe even Elle Macpherson too. But on the inside, I just felt tired.

Problem #2: **Monotony**. To people who don't understand it, I'm sure running looks like a very boring activity. That may be, but I'm positive it's ten times more interesting than walking. (At the very least, the scenery moves by more quickly.) Walking miles and miles can be best illustrated like this: left, right, left, right. Pleasant, wasn't that? Just multiply that by ten thousand and you'll quickly see what I mean.

Problem #3: **Heat**. Getting up early helped, of course. But once the endurance walks reached upwards of five or six hours long, the days were turning rather warm by the time I finished. At that point, I would stumble into my driveway like Clark Griswold emerging from the desert.

Problem #4: **Cars**. Nothing temporarily overcomes the tribulations associated with lack of ambition, monotony, and heat quite like one ton of steel whizzing by at fifty miles per hour just two feet from your left frontal lobe. It only took a couple weeks of this before I sought an alternate path.

A couple of days before the ten-mile practice day, I got in the car to plot out my course. The idea was simple: drive five miles from home, mentally mark the spot, and return home. Ta da! Ten miles, just like that. Now I'm not sure if this is general knowledge or not, but cars are capable of moving a *lot* faster than humans are.* I'm not sure I fully considered this, psychologically, as I prepped for the actual walk.

I woke up early Saturday and dressed. I packed plenty of water and set out. My goal was to finish in about two and a half hours. I don't remember now how long it actually took, but it felt more like two and a half days. It was nothing but *left, right, left, right, left, right, whiiiiiiizzzzzz, jump, left, right, left, right, left, right, stumble, right, right, left, right, left, right, whiiiiiiizzzzzz, jump, etc., etc., etc.* The miles passed slowly. I wouldn't have outrun a herd of turtles stampeding through peanut butter.

But I did make it through the day. Once I got home, I had a couple bowls of Honeycomb cereal with strawberries for breakfast and pondered my future. All I could think was *this was the easy walk. They're going to get longer, and longer, and longer.* I knew someday soon I would be wistfully looking back on the days where I "only" had to walk ten miles. The only thing that kept me from quitting altogether was the embarrassment of quitting altogether. I have to believe that's the only thing that kept Bruce Jenner going too.

Beth was going through similar trials. If I could have had one wish, it would have been the opportunity to do the workouts together. Well, that's not entirely true. If I could have had *one* wish, it would have been to win the Power Ball lottery jackpot. Then I could have paid someone else to do the workouts while I watched him via satellite. As it was, I didn't win the lottery, and Beth was still working out on her own, over three hundred miles to the east.

But there is good news in this story—something I think we're all ready for, if nothing more than to just to stop my incessant whining for two flippin' minutes. The more I walked, the eas-

---

* Well, humans costing less than six million dollars, that is.

ier the walking became. I know! It sounds crazy, doesn't it? The endurance weeks progressed to twelve, thirteen, fifteen, sixteen, and nineteen miles. I also re-routed my path to wind through quiet suburban neighborhoods, instead of long, dusty country roads punctuated by harrowing highway crossings. Everything really felt like it was coming together. The nineteen-mile day wasn't half as bad as that very first ten-mile day.

But then it unexpectedly got bad again. On the twenty-mile day, something came up and I wasn't able to walk at all. When it came time to do the twenty-one-mile day, I only completed twelve miles, due to time constraints. On top of all that, my mid-week walks weren't as consistent as they used to be. As the last days before the marathon closed in, I felt like I was taking a few steps backwards. Beth, too, had troubles keeping up with the program. (Life as a single mom added an extra layer of difficulty to her marathon training.)

But we weren't going to let any troubles keep us from our goal. We established a target for ourselves back in April and we were going to see it through no matter what. But, still, I'd be lying if I said I wasn't starting to doubt my ability to complete an entire marathon. Nineteen miles is good, but it left the 7.2 most difficult miles as completely uncharted territory.

Chapter 13

"Just for the Taste of It"

When I was about thirteen, I established a weekly ritual. My mom* would regularly buy Pepsi in glass bottle eight-packs. (If you're too young to remember buying soft drinks in these thick, heavy glass bottles, let me tell you, you really missed out.) While we were certainly aware of diet soft drinks at the time, we didn't honestly believe they were meant for human consumption.

My first introduction to diet sodas happened a few years earlier, when I dropped a quarter into a vending machine, pressed the COKE button, and a pink can of something called TAB rolled out. I had no idea what it was (and it *certainly* wasn't what I wanted) but it was a hot summer day, and I was thirsty. I popped the top, took a swig, and immediately spit it out. I couldn't imagine what sort of people thought kerosene was a reasonable substitute for a cold beverage. The rest of the family apparently shared my views, given that we continued to buy regular, sugar soda pop. We weren't concerned with extra calories, and considering an eight pack of

---

* Not her real name.

bottles weighed about twenty pounds, we worked off the extra calories just lugging them home from the store.

Each week, when the Pepsi supply was refreshed, I would nab one bottle to share amongst me, myself, and I. This bottle went into the basement fridge and stayed there until party-hard Friday night. This was my weekly reward for a punishing week of eighth grade.

If you're wondering how a geeky thirteen-year old with no friends partied hard each Friday, it went something like this:

6:00 PM. **Dinner Time**. If I was lucky, we had tacos. If I was *really* lucky, we had tacos on paper plates. (I don't know why paper plates made such a difference, but they did.) If I wasn't so lucky, it was slumgullion. I'm not sure if what *we* called slumgullion is what the rest of the world calls slumgullion, but that's beside the point. All I remember is it was made of ground beef, elbow macaroni, and big, wet chunks of tomatoes: hardly in my top ten. But the tacos! I wish I could go back in time and figure out how my mom made them. I know it was just ground beef cooked with pre-packaged seasonings, but what really put them over the edge is they were *fried*. After the meat went into corn tortillas, she'd dropped them in a shallow pan of boiling Wesson oil for a minute or two. Man, talk about a decadent meal. I could eat at least a dozen of those things in a sitting and not break a sweat.

6:50 PM. **Prep Time**. After dinner, I cleared the table, washed and dried the dishes, and put everything away. (Revisionist History Alert: I did none of that.) Um, I mean after dinner, once *someone else* had cleared the table, washed and dried the dishes, and put everything away, I would go downstairs to retrieve my semi-secret, icy cold bottle of high fructose corn syrup heaven. On the way back upstairs, I'd grab a box of Cheez-Its for some serious snackage. (Cheez-Its, by the way, are an incredible snack cracker. You'd be hard-pressed to find more crunchable goodness in a single square inch than the Cheez-It. And, no, Cheese Nips are *not* the same.) With refreshments in hand, I settled down in front of the television for an evening of CBS-provided bliss.

7:00 PM. **Science & Violence Time**. The evening began at seven o'clock with *The Incredible Hulk*. If there were ever a better show for the lonely junior high kid on a Friday night, I don't know what it was. If I ever write another book, I just might consider calling it *All I Really Need to Know I Learned from The Incredible Hulk*. What a way of life that guy had. He would typically go about minding his own business, when he'd suddenly find himself (or someone close to him) wronged or otherwise in trouble. At that point, he would get mad, turn green, toss a few bad guys around, then move on to the next town. For some reason Dr. Banner was always trying to find a way *out* of this life. What a moron. Thousands of kids would have traded body parts for this kind of lifestyle.

8:00 PM. **Stupid Time**. After an hour of intellectual stimulation provided by the jolly green giant, it was time to downshift, mentally speaking. What better way to do that than with Bo and Luke Duke? What a way of life those guys had. They would typically drive around minding their own business, find themselves (or someone close to them) wronged or otherwise in trouble. At that point, they would get even by racing the *General Lee* around the countryside and jumping it seventy feet through the air. (Even at a young age, I never failed to notice how the car's front end would be completely crushed upon landing, but somehow they just kept right on going.) Oh, and let's not forget Daisy Duke. If I decide against writing the aforementioned Hulk book, I may instead have to write *Everything I Need to Know I Learned from Catherine Bach's Wardrobe*.

9:00 PM. **Down Time**. Neither *Dallas* nor the ten o'clock news with Bill Kurtis and Walter Jacobson did anything for me, so I would be forced to take a ninety-minute break from the tube and do something else. It's really too bad we didn't have a VCR back then so I could watch old episodes of *The Incredible Hulk* or *The Dukes of Hazzard*. (Although, to be fair, Bill and Walter really *did* have the best news program there ever was. I should have watched it more when I had the chance. Today's news just isn't the same.)

10:30 PM. **Bed Time**. The television viewing evening wrapped up with re-runs of *The New Avengers*. With my Pepsi long gone and my stamina fading, I would typically fall asleep before I found out how the week's adventures concluded. Not that this mattered much, since I'd end up in a dream wearing John Steed's bowler and foiling the plot of a double agent with Purdey at my side.

So you can see I have many fond memories associated with carbonated, cola flavored, caramel colored sugar water. My love of the syrupy beverage continued throughout high school, college, and for some years after. I did, of course, try diet soft drinks from time to time—usually out of necessity due to lack of other choices. They still tasted like kerosene and I was positive that Coke's "just for the taste of it" motto really was "just for the marketing spin."

By late 1989 or early 1990, I began to realize that the empty calories needed to be dealt with. The easiest target was definitely these sugar-laden drinks. So with great reluctance I began buying diet soft drinks *on purpose*. I must admit, the conversion wasn't easy. They still tasted terrible, and I wondered what the point of the whole affair was. I mean, if you don't want to drink sugar sodas, just drink water, or iced tea, or something else. Why try to fake it? It makes no sense.

Diet soda is definitely an acquired taste. (Another one of life's mysteries I'll never understand. If you don't like a certain taste, why try it over and over again until you get to the point where you can tolerate it? Then, once tolerance is reached, continuing to tolerate it until you actually learn to like it?) But for whatever reason, I kept at it until a strange thing happened: I liked it. I actually *liked* it. It didn't taste funny. It didn't taste "diet" or artificial. It just tasted like soda. For a number of years, I equally liked both sugar and sugar-free sodas—probably the only person on earth with that rare condition. But after a time I eventually cut out the sugar sodas completely. It wasn't because of calories this time either. No, I actually preferred the diet soft drinks. Holy crap. I was drinking them just for the taste of it.

We can thank a man named Hyman Kirsch for diet drinks. He was a Russian immigrant living in Brooklyn who began selling soft drinks in 1904. Years later, he became involved with an institution known as the Jewish Sanitarium for Chronic Disease. The hospital's diabetic and heart patients were on sugar-restricted diets, for obvious reasons. Hyman, along with his son, developed a sugar-free drink that could be enjoyed by these particular patients. In 1952 their product, "No-Cal" brand soda pop was introduced. This unique, new beverage was a hit. Inviting flavors such as black cherry or chocolate* quickly created a devoted following. Their success didn't go by unnoticed. When Coke and Pepsi decided to take on this new market, No-Cal didn't stand a chance against the beverage behemoths and by the 1960s, Kirsch Bottling was out of the game. (I've since heard the company was resurrected in 2005. I really need to find some and try it.)

Diet sodas were initially sweetened with cyclamates, a chemical substance developed to literally "help the medicine go down"; Abbott Laboratories originally purchased the patent from DuPont to help soften the bitterness of antibiotics.

---

* That was the exact flavor, "Black Cherry or Chocolate."

Eventually it found its way into food products and beverages. I'm too young to have ever had a diet drink using this artificial sweetener. My entire memory of cyclamates is that of my dad's indignant complaints about the ban. Based on evidence that they caused bladder cancer in lab rats, the FDA banned cyclamates in 1969. What bugged him the most (and I'm not sure where his data came from) is that the rats were given something like the equivalent of four hundred bottles of diet soda a day. "If you give four hundred bottles of *anything* a day to an animal," he'd say, "it's going to develop problems."

But my dad and the other cyclamate proponents lost and the US was forced to convert to saccharin. Blecch. My first memory of this stuff was a product called *Sweet 10*. It was a clear liquid intended (in our house) to be squirted into coffee. I squirted some onto my tongue once and about gagged. How could something that was purported to be several hundred times sweeter than sugar could taste so awful? My second memory of saccharin was the aforementioned can of Tab. Blecch again. Like cyclamates, this artificial sweetener did bad things to rats too. Unlike the unlucky cyclamate, it was never officially banned. Instead, warning labels were required on products containing it. Eventually the proposed ban was lifted and the warning label requirement rescinded. Blecch.

By the time saccharin was "safe" again, it was too late. A new product had arisen to take its place. This time the yummy substance known as aspartyl-phenylalanine-1-methyl ester—or just Aspartame for short. Like cyclamates, it wasn't originally supposed to be an artificial sweetener. It was created while working on an anti-ulcer drug in 1965. It too went through a dead lab rat phase; but was ultimately approved for use in beverages in 1983. It rose to prominence under the brand name NutraSweet though it raised a few eyebrows with the scary warning to phenylketonurics that it contained phenylalanine. While this sounds like some creepy chemical compound, it's actually just a natural amino acid. (We talked about those back on page 103.) If you are still worried that you might have phenylketonuria and not know it, fear not: *you'd know it.* If you thought *your* last diet was restrictive, consider the unfortunate phenylketonuric. No meat of any kind, no fish, no nuts, no milk, cheese, or any other dairy product. So far so good, huh? Well, there's no bread, pasta, potatoes or corn either. If you've been happily eating any of these foods for more than a day or two, you needn't worry about the soda can warning.

Last up is sucralose, which you're more likely to recognize under its brand name Splenda. The little yellow packet has become all the rage in artificial sweeteners over the last few years. It was first created in 1975 and, like all the others, its use as a sweetener was a lab accident. Splenda's popularity stems from the fact that it does taste more like sugar and it is very heat stable, making it the ideal artificial sweetener for baking and cooking.

The marketing states it's "made from sugar so it tastes like sugar." This is technically true. It does enter the world as sucrose but three of the sucrose molecule's hydroxyl groups are swapped out for chlorine atoms. So, yes, chemically speaking Splenda contains chlorine. As you can well imagine, sugar producers aren't too happy with Splenda's "we're the same as sugar!" claims. There's nothing natural about it.

The other issue is that sucralose can't be easily used in its pure form. The stuff you find in the little yellow packets is bulked up with maltodextrin and glucose. For these reasons, Splenda is not calorie free: one cup contains nearly one hundred calories. (Compare to sugar, which has close to eight hundred.) However, since the individual packets clock in at under five calories, it's legal to call that "zero calories." (Say, I think the next time I gain five pounds, I'll claim the legal right to say I gained zero.)

Splenda is gaining ground in the market quickly. Many people prefer it to the other choices. When I first tasted it, I remember thinking it was pretty good. I was even happy when I first saw it used in soft drinks, thinking it might make them a bit closer to the real thing. Either my tastes have changed since then or something in the Splenda has changed because I just don't like it any more. Sodas made with it taste weird to me. A few weeks ago, I even tried some cheesecake made with Splenda. Each bite came with two distinct tastes: first the cheesecake, then the "sweetener." It was awful. It took me almost thirty seconds to finish the whole thing. (Well, it *was* cheesecake.) If I had a choice, though, I'd go with desserts made with NutraSweet. No, wait, I take that back. If I actually had a choice, I'd make it so real sugar didn't make me fat at all. Then I'd eat the real stuff all the livelong day.

But are artificial sweeteners safe? On the one hand, they've been with us for decades and consumed by tens of millions of people. If there were something seriously wrong with them, we would know by now, right? The answer to that depends on whom you ask. Because on the other hand, besides five more fingers, you have those who believe artificial sweeteners are responsible for every modern ill since the bubonic plague.* One would think something *that* dangerous would have been noticed by now. The answer to that, of course, is a gigantic cover-up. Now I love a good conspiracy as much as the next tinfoil-hat nut cake, but this just seems like a little too hard to believe.

Still, artificial sweeteners *are* artificial. Who's to say that something won't go wrong ten, fifty, or a hundred years from now? We could be horribly endangering ourselves and not yet know it. For all we now know, it could be worse than global warming. We may one day have to face the prospect of a movie where Dennis Quaid walks to New York to save his son from Splenda. So if you really, really, really want to be safe, then just avoid them at all costs. It seems like the most prudent thing to do.

But, man! They've become so much a part of my life that I can't imagine getting along without them. And believe me I've

---

* Perhaps even *including* the bubonic plague.

tried. I've made many attempts at giving up diet soda in favor or drinking more water. I *know* water's better for me. But, dang it, I *really like diet sodas*. Part of it is just for the taste of it, sure. But most of it is just for the way they bring all the little broken pieces of my life together into a coherent whole. Diet sodas complete me.

Chapter 14

A Walk in the City

In 490 B.C., King Darius of Persia attempted to conquer Greece and annex it to the Persian Empire. The Greeks were the underdogs but ultimately prevailed. Legend has it that an Athenian runner named Pheidippides ran from the battlefield near the town of Marathon to Athens to announce the victory. He ran the twenty-six mile trip without stopping, made his announcement, then promptly kicked the bucket. Thus, I cannot stress enough the importance of spending every Saturday the summer before the run building up endurance.

On Thursday, October 8, 1998, Beth called me up. We chatted about how things were going and whether or not we were ready for the big day. She mentioned that she hadn't had as much time to train lately. I confessed that things had not been going well for me either. She also said she felt like she had a bit of a cold. I felt fine, if a bit nervous. Still, we were still in good spirits and had high hopes for a successful day.

I drove to Chicago as planned on Friday. She took the day off to rest. But by Saturday morning, she wasn't getting any better. She still had a cough but now also complained of tightness in her chest. We finally convinced her to go see the doctor. Some hours later, my mom and I were upstairs in her home office where she'd enlisted me for some PC repair work. Somehow she always managed to save up computer-related problems for my visits—just one of the many dangers of being ~~a geek~~ a good son. Anyway, while I was replacing a CD-ROM drive (which, by the way, does not double as a cup holder) Beth's six-year old daughter came up stairs with a matter-of-fact report, delivered in her halting six-year old voice, "My mom just got home from the doctor and she's crying because she has bronchitis and can't do the marathon tomorrow."

I believe the doctor's words were, "A marathon? *Tomorrow*? Yeah, right."

Needless to say, Beth was a bit upset. And angry. And frustrated. The months of planning, training, fund-raising—*everything*—all of that completely dashed to pieces. Beth had not been sick in years, and now this: kicked out just one day before the big event.

The evening before the race I pulled my gear together, trying to make sure everything would be ready to go first thing in the morning. I'd felt briefly elated earlier in the day when we picked up our race packets, but that high was now long gone. The sobering fact before me now was: I was going to walk the Chicago Marathon alone. This wasn't right. This wasn't the plan at all. *Beth* was going to walk the marathon with the Team in Training group. This was *her* goal. I was just the tag-along.

"I know," I thought to myself, around eleven that night, "I'll call Jenn and see if she's doing anything tomorrow."

"Hello?" she picked up the phone, sleepily. I could actually hear her rubbing her eyes.

"Hey, it's me. Beth's sick and can't walk the marathon in the morning. Do you want to go with me?"

"Do I need to train or anything?" she asked.

"Nah, it's easy. Just a few laps around the block."

"Really?"

"Really!" I assured her.

"Um, okay..."

So the next morning Jenn and I headed down to the race together and she ended up giving me a piggyback ride for the full twenty-six miles. It was the best day of my life.

And that's when I woke up. It was about four in the morning, a good two hours before the race. I slept fitfully for maybe another hour, before crawling out of my nice, warm bed. I dressed, assembled my belongings, and made ready to depart.

While packing the previous evening, it dawned on me that I didn't have any of the actual details worked out. I didn't know what time I needed to leave, or where I would park, or if I would even know where to go once I got downtown. No wonder I didn't sleep well.

As I fumbled about, Laura suddenly offered to drive me downtown and drop me off. Of course! What an obvious solution. What made me think I had to do this all on my own?

This temporary high quickly dissipated as we drove down the Eisenhower expressway toward the lake in the early five o'clock hour. I was tired—more tired than I should be before such an event. I also felt fat. Unbelievably, after a summer of intense marathon training and watching what I was eating, my weight didn't drop much more than a few more pounds. All told, I was still over two hundred. True, I was probably in my best shape since 1991. It was just depressing now to discover that my best shape was "fat."

Laura dropped me off somewhere within a hundred yards or so of where I needed to be. It was dark. I took off my sweats and threw them in the back of the car. I felt cold. We said our good-byes and she drove off. There I stood, like an idiot. For the life of me, I couldn't understand what I was doing there. This was a race for skilled long-distance runners; not overweight walking tag-alongs who couldn't even point to the starting line.

My only plan at this point was to locate the Team in Training group and figure out a way to blend in. I didn't even think to grab her jersey. (Man, what was with my brain?) I guess I somehow still expected Beth to be wearing it and standing next to me. Instead, she was home and in bed* while I was looking for a group of people I didn't know, hoping I could slip in unnoticed, all the time worried about a tap on the shoulder saying, "Hey buddy, who the heck are you?"

Following the noise and lights to the starting area, I found I blended right in. No one took any notice of me over any other participant. There was a moderately large crowd too. It was hard to estimate, but I would guess at least two hundred. Moreover, there were all shapes and sizes represented. I was somewhat relieved to discover I wasn't the only person who looked like—well, a regular person. As I looked around, I realized at this very moment it wasn't about how much I weighed, how much I lost, or even how much I had left to lose. It wasn't about how much weight everyone else lost either. Who cares if we lost five pounds or five hundred pounds getting here? The fact was *we were here*. I felt a little better. Not much, but a little.

Around five minutes before six, they herded us over to the starting line. I somehow found myself near the front of the pack—a spot I *definitely* did not want. I quickly stepped aside and let others through the chutes as I eased my way towards the rear. It was still dark and cool and everyone was restless. Someone stood before the crowd, barking inaudible words through a bullhorn—most likely last-minute instructions or directions. I couldn't hear him at all, but it didn't matter. I was on the sheep plan: just follow the person in front of me.

The minutes passed slowly. At just a hair before six, the horn sounded and we pushed forward like cattle heading out to pasture (or slaughter). I heard someone off to my right exclaim with a thrill, "I can't believe it! This is actually happening!" Hey, my thoughts *exactly*.

---

* Hmmm...now that I think about it, probably on purpose.

Mile 1

It took no time at all for the large mass of bodies to stretch into a thin, straight line. My starting-gun high evaporated as that lonely, out-of-place feeling quickly returned. We walked a couple of blocks and soon found ourselves underground. One thing I couldn't train for was increased levels of pollution. The air in the lower passes wasn't exactly what I'd call refreshing. I had, after all, trained under the wide-open skies of Iowa farmland. Fortunately, that only lasted a few minutes, and we soon re-emerged at street level.

Most walkers broke off into small groups of two to four people. There were a few larger groups and very few singles. Perhaps walking all by oneself is not a very good idea.

After what seemed like at least an hour, the very first mile marker appeared. A woman behind me shouted, "Yay! There's Mile One," followed by stone silence. She quickly asked, "Am I the only one excited by that?" which made me laugh to myself. I checked my stopwatch. We were exactly seventeen minutes into the race.

Yes, *seventeen* minutes to walk one mile. I know, I know. It's rather pathetic. While I was certainly capable of walking quicker than that, I still had no idea what the full twenty-six miles would be like. All I had to go on were the three goals I had set for myself:

1. Finish.
2. Finish on my own two feet.
3. Finish on my own two feet before the course closed.

I had no intention of ending up as one of those *Agony of Defeat* athletes—crawling on hands and knees, gasping for breath, with city traffic hot on my heels. A nice, inconspicuous finish is what I had rather planned. No pictures of me in the morning *Tribune* necessary, thank you.

So for all these reasons, I had planned a 17:10 pace. This was more than comfortable for me and had the excellent property of working out to exactly seven and a half hours: the precise point when the course closed. So after only one mile, I was already ten seconds ahead of schedule. Woot!

Mile 2

We were still very much downtown at this point. When I got a peek through the buildings, I could see the eastern sky at last turning blue. I wasn't feeling any less out of place yet, either. The thought again crept into my head, "What on earth am I doing? Am I actually trying to complete a marathon?" Then here, at only twenty-five minutes into the race, the unthinkable entered my head. *I might not be able to finish this.* This was soon followed by the realization that I had no idea how to quit even if I wanted to. What would I do? Just hobble over to the curb, crawl up into a ball, and wait for the buzzards?

Miles 3 & 4

Shortly after the second mile marker, the course turned north for a long, five-mile march. It was also a turning point for me. I finally began to fall into stride. The sky brightened quite a bit and the buildings fell off as we put downtown Chicago to our heels.

By the fourth mile marker, I was implausibly ahead of my pace. I thought about slowing down, but didn't (in spite of the fact that the number one mistake of first-time marathoners is going too quickly too early). But I felt fine, and figured, *Hey, if it's a common trap, why not fall for it?* Plus, most of the other walkers were way ahead of me now and only a small few behind me. I consciously decided to keep up the pace.

Miles 5 & 6

The course drew near Lake Michigan where a brilliant orange sun, just peering out over the water, greeted us. It was beautiful. I couldn't have timed it better. We walked along a canal where a few dozen people fished, then followed a trail filled with the usual Sunday-morning exercisers. An older couple ahead saw the crowd gathered around the aid station near Mile Six and asked a pair ahead of me if that's where the walkers finished. "Nope, we're going the whole twenty six!" The couple seemed astonished, and with good reason. Walking the marathon *does* seem a bit crazy given our snail's pace.

I, on the other hand, no longer felt crazy. Nor did I feel out of place. Gone were all doubts and concerns. At mile marker six, I'd really found my place and let me tell you, that place felt pretty darn good. *This* is what I'd hoped it would be like. As I passed the marker I thought, "Hey, I'm nearly a quarter done!"

Miles 7 & 8

It was 7:42 AM and the official race was about to start six miles behind me. The course was now rapidly filling up with spectators. It's amazing what an incredible boost that is. The seventh mile went very well with the tremendous help of the ever-growing crowds.

Our northerly journey concluded at the end of this mile. We turned left and walked west for a couple blocks, then turned left again and looked south. I couldn't believe how far away the city appeared. I would have sworn the Sears Tower was thirty miles away. The thought once again crept back: *I might not be able to finish this.*

While strolling toward mile marker eight, I happened to notice I was now only two blocks west of mile marker six. "Dang!" I thought to myself. "I sure could have saved myself a good chunk of time there."

Just kidding. Cheating never entered my mind.

Sort of.

Mile 9

Near the beginning of this mile the first wheelchair entrants whizzed by. Now *these* athletes are amazing. I don't think I can begin to describe them other than to say they have more muscle in one arm than I have in my entire body. At only a half hour or so into the race, they'd already completed eight miles. If I'm right in my reckoning, that's about sixteen miles per hour: far ahead of anyone on foot. Wow.

Halfway into the ninth mile we hit Clark and took the diagonal street on a slow southeasterly course. A group of cheerleaders decked out in short skirts and pompons greeted us enthusiastically. They were hot too, as long as your definition of "hot" includes hairy legs, beer bellies, cheap wigs and full beards.

A quarter of a mile later, the frontrunners passed. There was a cavalcade of official cars, motorcycles and police plowing the way, followed by the camera crews and lastly the pace car. My jaw dropped when I saw the race clock. The last mile, it announced, was run in 4:47. If they maintained this pace, the winner might actually set a new world record. And there was quite a tight pack of them too.

If I didn't know any better, I would have said they weren't human. They were machines. Feet pounded the pavement rhythmically, almost mechanically; heads upright and eyes focused, arms pumping. I can't imagine in my wildest dreams running one mile in less than five minutes and here was a fair-sized group of people about to run twenty-six of them. It just didn't seem possible.

Miles 10, 11 & 12

After ten miles, my thoughts drifted back to the *Dam to Dam* race. On that day at this point, I was tired and more than ready for the race to be finished. Today, I was still going strong and (surprisingly) still gaining on my anticipated time. "I sure have come a long way in just four months," I thought.

As I strode toward the eleven-mile mark, we crossed the river one more time and followed it for a couple blocks as it curved towards Wacker Drive. A live band played and spectators absolutely packed the course, many bodies deep. It was almost overwhelming at points. In fact (and this may sound strange) I felt a little embarrassed that I wasn't running. It's hard to describe. Perhaps by just walking, I didn't feel deserving of this kind of cheering by these kinds of crowds.

As I closed in on the twelve-mile mark, I began to get hungry. I wore a fanny-pack* and had stuffed it the day before with various supplies, including a cereal bar and two Pop-Tarts. I ate the cereal bar and continued.

I also began scanning the crowd for any signs of my own personal cheering section. I'd given the family a course map and labeled the times I expected to be at various points in the course. Since I was ahead of my own schedule, I worried we might miss each other.

Miles 13, 14 & 15

During the thirteenth mile, I passed the 20K marker. Memories of the June race flooded back a second time. "If this was then, I'd be done!" It was odd to think back on how twenty kilometers was such a big deal at the time. Yet by the end of my summer training, I actually looked *forward* to the twelve-mile days because they were so short.

At the halfway point, a large balloon rainbow arched over the course. The ChampionChip detectors beeped steadily as hundreds of feet galloped by.

"The halfway point," I pondered, but it can hardly be called that since the first half is the *easy* half. I probably had at least seventy percent of the course to go, from an expenditure point of view. I plodded on, continuing to scan the crowds for any signs of my supporters.

Mile 16

This was my first "worst" mile. It started when I crossed mile marker fifteen and ended about two weeks later. I wasn't tired and I wasn't sore, but for some reason it just *would not end*. Part of what made it so bad is that for the past few miles I couldn't help but feeling I was getting *farther* away from the

---

* They were having a sale down at The Gap.

finish line. Every time I felt the course had finally straightened out (you know, pointing toward the *end* of the race) we'd suddenly veer off in some other direction, clearly adding several more miles to the journey.

I was almost sure I'd lost the course and was wandering around downtown Milwaukee, when I looked ahead and saw those big yellow numbers: 1 and 6. Finally! My pleasure was doubled when I glanced up again and saw waving hands belonging to familiar faces. There they were! My fans! I was surprised to see them at all since I was nearly eleven minutes ahead of my pace. My daughter Sarah and niece Hannah stood on the edge of the road, arms stretched out and slapping runners' hands as they passed. Laura was there with the video camera and my mom had a fresh supply of snacks. I didn't need nor want any food at that point (having just finished one of the two aforementioned Pop-Tarts). They walked along with me for a couple dozen yards before the current whisked me off again.

Miles 17, 18 & 19

The seventeenth mile felt like it lasted two minutes, which more than made up for the previous "mile." Not only that, the course turned east again, which was always good for my spirits. Somehow, heading toward the city always felt like the "right" direction.

Not long into this mile, the family car passed by off to the right, as my fan club headed for the next rendezvous point. "Now I know why cars were invented," I mused.

Most of this section of the course took us through Little Mexico. The wonderful smells from the restaurants and bakeries was almost torture. It seemed a cruel twist of fate that so much of the course wound through neighborhoods like this. A funny picture flashed through my mind of a stream of runners diverted through restaurants, returning to the course, a taco in each hand. Actually, that might be a great race. The winner is declared by both time run and tacos eaten.

Mile 20

Crossing the nineteenth marker and starting the twentieth mile was a significant personal event. I thought *this is it: from here on out is all unknown territory*. I'd never gone farther than this during training.

While training, I would occasionally stop for water or even just to wiggle my toes. Today I had not stopped even once. The fact is I was afraid to. I was convinced that if I stopped walking, I'd never be able to start up again. I pushed aside all thoughts of rest (and bathroom breaks) and just focused on three things: moving, moving, and moving.

Fortunately, it was easier to keep moving during a real race. The crowds continued to cheer us on, a reggae band played, a woman shouted, "You can do it!" Although I had to ask the person next to me, "How does *she* know?"

We headed into Chinatown where a dancing Dragon greeted us. Drums and cymbals rang loudly as the runners (and walkers) funneled into the district. Spectators closed in tightly on the course, which I took as a sign that I was falling near the end of the pack.

Mile 21

The hopeful turn east we made during the nineteenth mile was short-lived. Much to my dismay, the course took another "wrong" turn and we were once again walking away from the finish line. This mile ended at Comiskey Park where I again considered calling Jenn for that piggyback ride.

My fan club greeted me once again. Sarah asked if I was done walking yet. (I certainly wished so.) Laura offered me a drink of her root beer. (I declined, not wanting to throw up just then and there.) My mom again inquired whether I wanted anything else to eat. (Nope.)

Believe it or not, I was still doing well—tired, of course, but still going sure and steady. My lower back was a bit sore, but my legs (and knees!) didn't hurt the way I'd expected. I had assumed that by this time I'd be lying on the curb waiting for emergency roadside assistance. Oddly enough, I was actually *passing* a few people. This was undoubtedly due to the fact that I was squarely in the midst of the end-of-the-packers, so shuffling places amongst the other slowpokes wasn't extraordinary. After the race, my mom commented how much different (read: worse) participants looked at this point than at mile sixteen: two markers which were a lifetime apart for some of us. The course continued south from here on the west side of the Dan Ryan expressway.

Mile 22

"Why couldn't Pheidippides have died *here*?"

This was a long one. This made that never-ending sixteenth mile look like a hundred-yard dash. One factor contributing to my dismal condition was watching racers on the east side of the Dan Ryan moving north. I couldn't see ahead where we crossed the expressway and began our final northward turn, but I knew it had to be close. Meanwhile, it was torture watching the racers who'd already completed the last major course turn.

Another factor was the heat. Sure, any normal person would have deemed this beautiful sunny day in early October simply wonderful—but we weren't normal. To a marathon participant, moving miles and miles through temperatures in the mid-70s feels like a trek through Death Valley. Cooler is definitely better.

I pulled out my second Pop-Tart. Up ahead there was a spectator on the sidelines shouting most enthusiastically. He was twenty-something, wearing khaki shorts, a sweatshirt, standard-issue Ray Bans, and a ball cap. He was clapping and yelling at the top of his lungs.

"Come on! Move it! You can do it! Let's go! You're the *real* marathoners! You're the Five Hour People! Come on...!"

He spotted my Pop-Tart wrapper and pointed.

"Look at *this* guy! He's eatin' a *cheeseburger*! You're the ones! You can do it! Move!"

Not long after that, the course finally hit its southernmost point. We turned east, crossed the expressway, and headed north. FINALLY. It felt so good. The sun was at my back, we were moving the right direction, and I was still conscious.

Mile 23

At the beginning of this mile, spectators shouted their support with chants of, "ONLY FOUR MORE MILES!" This news lifted my spirits a bit as first but then I quickly thought, "What do they mean *only*?" That's well over an hour of grief for a waddler like me. My ten-minute lead had now shrunk to five minutes. I was definitely slowing down and I still had four of the longest miles of my life ahead of me.

The aid stations began to hand out bananas. As much as I like the squishy fruit, I couldn't help but wonder: had none of the organizers ever watched a cartoon? I mean, what is the quintessential object used to make people slip and fall flat on their backs? I nearly wiped out twice slogging through what looked like the horrible wreck of a produce delivery truck.

Miles 24 & 25

"Will it ever end?" (I'm sure you're thinking the same thing. Believe me this is by design. The race was a pain to walk. It should be a pain to read about too.) Fortunately, (for both of us) the end is in sight. I was briefly refreshed by the sight of lake again and when I turned north on Lake Shore Drive, but the distances between each mile marker stretched out like I never thought possible. Miles sixteen and twenty-two now comparatively felt like a ride on a bullet train.

The thinning spectators continued to shout the standard words of encouragement. *Only two more miles! You've made it this far! You can do it!* The thinning participants responded with weak smiles and not-so-high fives. We trudged on mindlessly toward our elusive goal.

Me, I still hadn't stopped once. My earlier visions of cheeseburgers had long since been replaced with visions of port-a-potties. But I knew if I stopped now, not only would I not be able to get going again, I might not even regain consciousness. The sun was still hot. The pavement seemed endless. My legs were numb, my back was sore, and my feet and hands were swollen. I had been moving constantly now for nearly seven hours. I think my butt was still back at mile marker twenty-two.

Mile 26

The long twenty-fifth mile ended just past the McCormick Place tunnel. I didn't know it was a tunnel. I just figured I'd finally blacked out for good. But as my eyesight returned and I emerged from the darkness, I passed the next mile marker. Thus began the last (full) mile of the course. The spectators shouted, "Only one more mile to go!" but they couldn't have been more wrong. "No," I told myself weakly, "only one more mile *and three hundred and eighty five yards* to go." There's a big difference, you know.

The course plodded north and then jutted west a bit towards traffic. Cars honked as they passed, until it became utterly annoying. I walked passed two parked ambulances on my right and had half a mind to ask one of the drivers, "Does this bus go to Grant Park?"

I'm not sure if it was by oversight or outright malice, but the course designers saw fit to put a long, steep incline right near the end of the race. I don't think Everest-climbers ever had it this bad. In all reality, it was just a short on-ramp to Lake Shore Drive, but it made me immediately thankful that Chicago hosts one of the flattest marathon courses. I don't think I would have been able to finish a marathon in a full three dimensions.

Then just over the crest, I at last spied those long-awaited magical numbers: 2 and 6. And just three hundred eighty five yards past *that*: the finish line.

Mile 26.2

My original goal, as you may remember, was to finish in seven and a half hours. When I pulled ahead of my expected pace halfway through the race, I even fantasized of finishing in seven hours flat. The last few miles dashed that dream to pieces, but at least I was still moving.

Only a couple hundred more yards now. "Just keep moving. Don't pass out. Ignore your legs. You can go back and pick up your butt later. There are cheeseburgers and port-a-potties in your near future."

The mind reels as the finish line approaches. The whole day—no, entire *months*—are at last coming to a decisive close. Only some dozens of yards ahead: a large sign. I think I can make out the word *FINISH*. Ahhh...the sweet release is near!

I turn to look behind and can hardly believe my eyes. There are still people *behind* me. True, they probably started at 7:45 AM and not six, but I didn't care. I was going to finish and I wasn't going to be the last one. "I won't be in the paper tomorrow morning! Yay!"

I'm now just a few strides from the finish.

I mentally count it down.

"Three, two, one ... *DONE!*"

I glance at my stopwatch: *seven hours, thirty minutes, and thirty-five seconds*. Holy crap, would you look at that! I missed my target by just *half a minute*.

After the Race

Do you know what the main difference is between walking a marathon and running a marathon? When you cross the finish line running, you get to *stop* running. When you cross the finish line walking, you have to keep on walking. "And you thought you were done! Ha ha! No such luck, buddy."

The chute steered participants to several points: a spot to turn in your ChampionChip, another spot to get your medal. (A medal! I had no idea! I thought those were reserved for people who finished the same day they started.) And still another spot beyond that for blankets. (Blankets?)

But it seemed to go on and on and on. All I wanted to do was *stop walking*. You know, just *end the race*. Continuing to walk, I suddenly found myself in what looked like a farmers market. More bananas, apples, bagels, and—hey, what's that?—a Samuel Adams truck tapping kegs and giving out beer! It would have been a welcome sight if I hadn't just spent the entire day on an asphalt treadmill.

I passed the beer truck with mixed emotions and at last saw a familiar face; my mom spotted me and waved. I hobbled over and found Laura and the girls there too, cameras rolling. I was hoping to see them all at the finish line, but that can be a real trick to pull off without a homing device.

I couldn't believe the ordeal was over. Heck, I couldn't believe I actually finished it. I tried to imagine what other participants felt as they crossed the finish line. It seemed likely that most would feel an enormous sense of accomplishment. They would feel like they were on top of the world. They'd be bursting with pride. I don't have to imagine what I felt. I remember it as if it were yesterday: *what a colossal waste of time*. Seriously. My mind flooded quickly with the memories of countless hours practicing. Weeks and months gone by just like that, never to be recovered. All for a walk in the city on one fine autumn Sunday. I hate to sound cynical, but I can't lie. That's what I was thinking.

The strange thing is, a marathon is not supposed to be a big deal. Human beings, anthropologically speaking, are in fact very good at long distances. I may have completed 26.2 miles today, but so did about seventeen thousand other people. Annually, upwards of half a million people in the US alone complete marathons. Jenn, her husband, and many of his siblings routinely run them. And then there are hikers all over the world who walk *at least* twenty-six miles a day for months and months on end. So not only did I feel like I'd wasted all that time training, it was all for something that really shouldn't be that remarkable. I came in last place out of the several million other people that came before me.

But for the moment, everyone else was proud and happy, so I went along. My mom said she was inspired to start exercising again, and asked me if I thought she could do next year's marathon. I replied with a quick *no*. Not because I didn't believe she could, but because I felt it was now my duty to deter all other humans from attempting this. It was for her own good, after all.

She then asked if I'd do another one. I shook my head, of course. But do you want to hear something insane? A small voice in a tiny corner of my mind said, "Hmmm... maybe."

"Just maybe..."

But not this week.

The walk to the car was absolutely excruciating. On the drive home rigor mortis set in. I was barely able to pull myself out of the car and up the porch steps. That last ten yards was worse than the previous four miles.

Once inside I collapsed in a chair and pulled off my shoes and socks. OH MY! You have *no* idea how good that felt. Simply wonderful. Utterly indescribable. I wiggled my doggies as they all breathed a collective sigh of relief.

A short while later my cheeseburger dream came true when Laura showed up with a couple of White Castle bags. I downed perhaps a dozen sliders and slipped off to sleep.

And that's my lesson for you today. If someone ever comes up to you and asks, "Cheeseburgers or a marathon?" you say, *cheeseburgers*.

I'm not joking.

Chapter 15

How to Start Your Own Diet Craze

There's only one thing better than losing weight and that's making piles of money off of it. I can think of no better way of doing that than by starting your own diet craze. Considering the thousands of people who've done this over the last century, it really can't be that hard. Although I've never started one myself,* I have a good inkling of how to go about it.

The most important part of any craze is that it *has* to work. If it doesn't, you'll just end up on the wrong side of a class action lawsuit and no one wants that. So how do you make sure your diet can't fail? Easy: make sure it's based on either exercising more or eating less (preferably both, if you can manage it). After all, this is the *only* way to guarantee weight loss, so why even bother looking for anything else?

The next two steps are: 1) cleverly disguise the eating right and/or exercising system so customers don't recognize that that's what's *really* going on; and 2) make an infomercial. When it comes to disguising your program, you luckily have a wide assortment of options at your disposal.

---

* I've been too busy watching television.

The Exercise Route

If your new craze is primarily based on exercising, then you **must** make sure the exercising looks **fun**. You simply cannot advertise participants grimacing and wincing the whole way through. (Never mind that in real life exercising isn't fun and certainly involves disagreeable facial expressions.) But for your product's success, it's paramount that your exercises look effortless.

Inventing an exercise-based craze starts with choosing one of two basic approaches: 1) moving around a lot; or 2) inventing a new machine. If you can somehow pull off #1, then I highly recommend going that route. You'll have lower startup costs and no expensive inventories to maintain. If you're forced to take the second route, then your costs will be far higher, but the payoff can be much larger if your margins are wide enough.

If you choose the "moving around a lot" approach, you have to find a known fitness guru, a former athlete, or at least a good B- or C-list celebrity. It helps a lot if this person is in shape too. (Not to mention it's a *real* bonus if he or she wasn't in shape at all a year or two ago.) Once your spokesperson has been booked, get a TV studio, a group of seven hot female models, two male models, and some upbeat music. Put the women in front, the two token guys way in the back, and roll camera. As long as they're jumping around and sweating to some up-tempo music, you've got it made. The last thing you need is a handful of testimonials. Interview at least a half dozen people and get them to tell you how jumping around and sweating to some up-tempo music changed their lives. Don't bother interviewing anyone who hasn't lost at least thirty pounds. If you can get triple digit weight losses, all the better.

The "inventing a new machine" approach will require inventing a new machine, of course. That's the tough part. But as long as it's something that has "abs" in the name, you're virtually guaranteed to strike gold. People *love* machines that work their abs. Once you've invented the machine, you will need some computer-generated graphics that demonstrate how the technology works. Important: Make sure the graphics look like a blueprint. That's how customers will know your machine is very technical in nature. After all, if it's technical, it has to work. Also, make sure that you show a computerized wire frame model of a fat person shrink down to a supermodel in just a few seconds. This will seal the deal.

The Eating Better Route

Like exercising, a food-based program also comes in two basic flavors: 1) a revolutionary new diet plan or 2) a revolutionary new diet pill.

The first option is the easiest, because all revolutionary new diet plans are the same. Just copy the last one, slap a new name on it, and hire a new pseudo-celebrity endorser. In case you can't remember what a program like this looks like, here's a quick run-down. A new program:

- Tells you why everything you know is wrong.
- Explains how this new approach is *The One.*
- Clarifies that it is not a fad.
- States you can eat all your favorite foods.
- Declares you don't have to change your lifestyle.

You must hit all these bullet points or you're doomed. My personal favorite is eating all your favorite foods ("and the pounds will just melt away!") This isn't a lie, mind you. You *can* eat all your favorite foods. The only trick is you have to eat microscopic portions of said foods. The snack industry has recognized a market for this and created the "One Hundred Calorie Snack Pack." They're all the rage now, especially among people needing external help in portion control. On the upside, it's good to have pre-sized portions at hand, rather than going through an entire Family Size bag in one sitting. On the downside, they're still just not-so-good-for-you snacks at a price easily more than double that of their Costco-sized counterparts. I tried the Doritos once. I thought, "Cool! Low calorie Doritos!" Imagine my disappointment when I found a bag of air with only two actual chips inside. I don't know about you, but I *love* Doritos. To me, a teeny tiny bag of them is punishment, not a treat. What am I to do? Probably eat six or seven of these little bags just to feel satisfied.

Anyway, back to our scheme. If you go with the "diet pill" option, you will have to invent some sort supplement. This may sound difficult, but don't worry, it's quite easy. All you have to do is toss together a bunch of all-natural herbs and give it a cool name, something like *Liponec AG 3000.* As an added bonus, because they're just herbs, there's no pesky FDA approval process to get in the way. If you don't know what kind to use, just pick any old tea out of the Far East, throw in some clover, and call it good. (Important: the farther away your herbs are from the United States, the better. Everyone knows domestic products aren't exotic, and therefore can't *possibly* work.)

Since you very well know your pill alone won't induce weight loss, you must come up with an accompanying low-calorie diet and exercise program. I recommend employing the one hundred calorie snack packs and sit-ups. Lastly, you're going to need some testimonials. Find people who've used your diet plan and/or herb, get good before-and-after photos, and let them tell their personal, inspiring stories.

Final Steps

Your infomercial is almost ready to air! You have two final steps. First, doctor endorsements are a must. Because your program is *really* just based on eating right and exercising, the doctors will *have* to agree that it will work. So getting the endorsement really just boils down to negotiating the exact height of the stack of Franklins. If the stack is high enough, you may even hit pay dirt by getting the doctor himself to tell everyone he's already tried it and lost twenty pounds.

Lastly, write your fine print. You'll never get anywhere without fine print (see the aforementioned class action lawsuit.) The fine print must state that your program alone won't get you anywhere at all. This is typically worded like so:

> "Participants lost weight using the Amazing Carbotastic Ab Trainer System™ combined with heavy exercise and a healthful, balanced, low-calorie diet. Your results, if any, will vary. RESULTS NOT TYPICAL."

And that's that! Go ahead and give it a shot. You can't possibly lose. Just remember, you owe me ten percent.

Chapter 16

Adrift

The Chicago Marathon marked the end of an era for me. It began in early 1997 when I embarked on a long-term walking program and ended in late 1998 with a bag of White Castle cheeseburgers. Through it all, I managed to lose 32 pounds. While this looks good on the surface, look at the details:

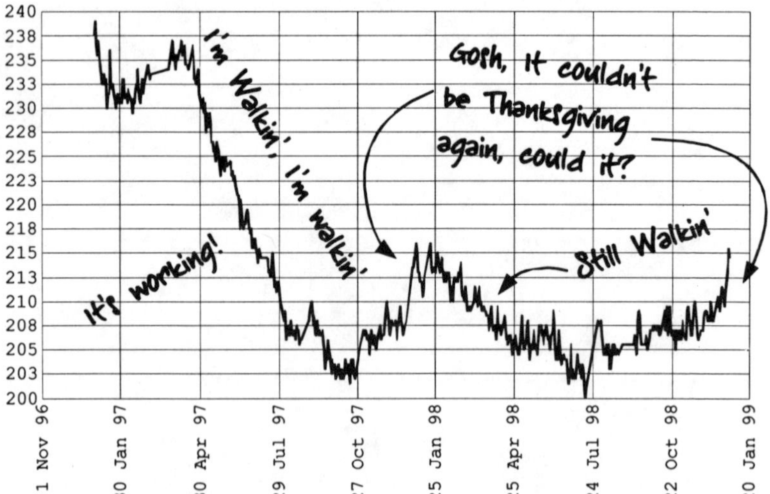

As you can see, at one point I was actually down by thirty-nine pounds. I continued to train but ironically *gained* weight between July and October. Most people will offer, "Yeah, but it's likely you were putting on muscle, and that weighs more than fat." That may have been true, but I sure didn't feel it. Not by a long shot.

After I returned to Des Moines, I told a co-worker about a photograph snapped of me during the race.

"How did you look?" she asked.

"Fat and slow," was my frank response.

We laughed, but it was true. When I started walking nearly two years earlier, my ultimate goal was to recapture the success I had in 1991, when I cracked the 170 mark. I truly believed that if I'd done it once as an adult then there was no reason I couldn't do it again. It was just a matter of hard work and perseverance. Yet here I was. All told, I'd walked about a thousand miles. Half of them were in the last six months alone. All that and I *still* couldn't even get my weight below two hundred pounds. It was a cold, hard slap in the face.

Now at this point one would think that I would give up. After all, I had a double whammy: 1) I fell short of my goal by more than thirty pounds; and 2) the holidays were on the way. But I didn't give up. For some reason, I kept trying. I did a little more walking. I tried a little weight lifting in the basement. I did some stretching and calisthenics—nothing serious and nothing that stuck.

In early November, Stephanie told me about a weight loss system she'd seen on an infomercial and decided to buy. The exercises looked strange, she told me, but the claims and testimonials appeared to be satisfactory and she figured *Oh, what the heck.* Apparently, all you had to do was breathe and the weight melted right off.

"You're kidding, right?" I asked incredulously.

"Nope, that's the way it works," she countered.

"All you do is *breathe*? How on earth does that work?"

"No idea," she stated flatly. "Do you want to give it a try?"

"Oh, what the heck," I said.

The system was called BodyFlex. It was being peddled by an attractive fifty-something woman named Greer Childers. If you haven't already seen the program yourself, I'm not quite sure if my explanations will do it justice.

The basic idea is to get more oxygen moving through your system. Most people are shallow breathers, pumping only the barest minimum of oxygen through their lungs and bloodstreams. Greer claims this oxygen deprivation keeps people from losing weight. If only you can get past this block, the pounds will melt away.

I popped the tape in the VCR. She demonstrated the basic technique. First, breathe out slowly, emptying your lungs as much as possible without passing out. Next, fill your lungs extremely quickly by gulping massive volumes of air through your nose. Lastly, return the air to the earth's atmosphere by means of a violent exhaling technique.

For some reason, she calls this system "BodyFlex." I guess that's because no one would buy a weight loss program called "Suck 'n' Blow." Granted, you *are* supposed to execute this breathing technique in a variety of oddly named positions.* The calisthenics do help you stretch out and get more flexible but it's obvious the emphasis is *definitely* on the breathing.

I probably did it for a week before giving up. The hardest part was just finding time when there wasn't another human within a quarter mile radius because I *sure* didn't want anyone seeing me do it. I also began to wonder if the product's claims were a little too good to be true. Sure enough, they were. In 2003, a lawsuit was filed by the FTC for false or unsubstantiated claims. The case was settled a year later in favor of the FTC. The defendants had to pay $2.6 million in refunds to people who were promised they'd lose between four

---

* Including everyone's favorite, "The Cat."

and fourteen inches in just seven days without changing their caloric intake. As of today, Greer is still in business. The program is essentially the same; they've just corrected the claims and adjusted the now all too familiar fine print:

> TYPICAL RESULTS ARE 4.8 INCHES LOST ACROSS 6 BODY PARTS IN 14 DAYS. RESULTS BASED ON FOLLOWING THE COMPLETE BODY FLEX EXERCISE AND DIET PROGRAM. BODY FLEX PROGRAM IS DEEP BREATHING, EXERCISE AND 1600 CALORIE PER DAY MEAL PLAN.

So let's see if I got this straight. If you exercise regularly and limit your caloric intake, you're going to lose weight? It's a miracle! How did she ever come up with something like that? Sarcasm aside, though, it's not a bad system. *No* system is bad that encourages you to eat better and move around a bit. It just annoys me that they constantly bury this stuff in the fine print. (But that's better than no fine print at all, as the FTC will tell you.)

The next two years turned out to be an utter mess. As I scan through my notes from the period, I had more than a dozen "Day One" marks on the calendar. Every time around it was the same sad dance:

1. I'd reach some new weight.
2. I'd get frustrated over it.
3. I'd screw myself up for another go.
4. I'd lose a few pounds.
5. Something bad like donuts would happen.
6. I'd have to start all over.

Worse, the "start over" point was always greater than the previous starting weight. It was like watching high tide roll in, each set of waves crashing higher than before. But it was also quite *unlike* watching the tide roll in. Because at least with the tide you know that twelve hours later it's going to roll right back out. For me, every twelve hours just ushered in yet another even higher tide.

You know, you'd think after losing upwards of a thousand pounds and gaining it all back again, reality would sink in at some point. The intelligent and rational person would face up to the facts and realize that *this just isn't working*. This person would give up and move on with his life. I've heard it said that the definition of insanity is doing the same thing over and over again and expecting different results. My behavior definitely fit this pattern. I'm sure scientists studying me like a lab rat would by now have killed and dissected me to discover the source of the abnormal degeneration.

Heck, there were times I actually did feel like a lab rat. One of the worst aspects of any diet is not being able to find anything suitable to eat. So, like a rat in a cage, I'd head to the fridge and stare for a while. Finding nothing, I'd turn to the pantry. Nothing there either. How about the cupboard? Nope, still nothing. Well, how about the fridge? I'd endlessly circle the room, never finding the cheese. Sad, really.

Anyway, I believe this next graph says it all:

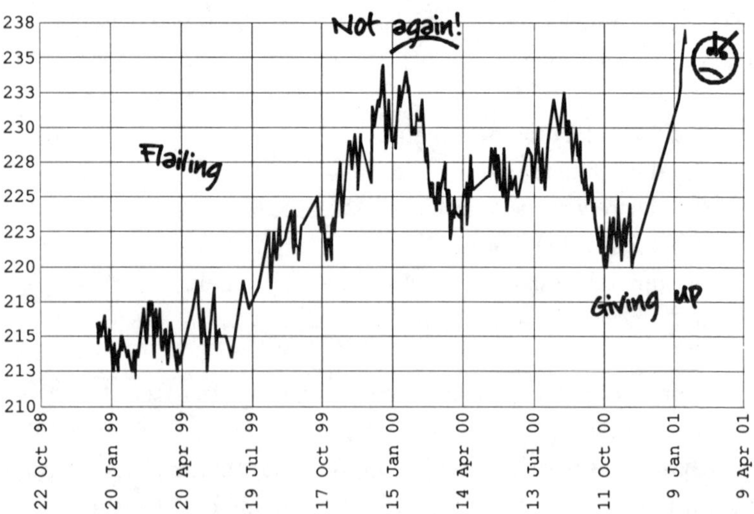

Clearly, something was seriously wrong. Things were wrong on so many levels. The 170 goal was at least one light-year away. I never even got close to 200. I gained seventeen pounds in the final two months alone—just two pounds shy of the all-time high. This was unimaginable no matter how I looked at it.

Nothing was working.

Nothing stuck.

The Switch was off and I was doomed.

At this point, I realized it was time for drastic measures. It was time for a completely new direction. It was time to turn the page and start a new chapter in my life.

Chapter 17

A New Chapter in My Life

In early 2000, while still adrift, one of my many attempted strategies was cutting down on my carb intake. I began to hear about how excess carbohydrates were to blame for all our ills and that eliminating them from the diet was a surefire way to lose weight. It sounded downright strange to me, but I was well acquainted with the principle of "excess" so I decided at least a *little* moderation was in order. I wrote:

> I'm starting to take control of the eating...mostly cutting down on carbohydrates and crap. It's not a full-blown high-protein, no-carb fad.

I didn't know the first thing about said full-blown, high-protein, no-carb fad. All I knew is that it sounded drastic and I wasn't quite ready for anything radical. After all, I'd always been able to lose weight before on traditional diets. (Never mind that I invariably gained it all back.)

But as you've now seen, the rest of 2000 did not go well. The time for drastic measures had definitely arrived. It was time to do some research.

Still intrigued by the idea of carb control, my research began with a book entitled *Dr. Atkins' New Diet Revolution*. Yes, that's right: Atkins. Oh, dear, where do I start with this? I can't think of a weight loss plan that has caused more controversy (or more sheer nuttiness, for that matter) than this one. Not only that, it's gone on for decades now. Most people call it a fad diet, but what kind of "fad" goes on for over thirty years?

I'm about to make a hypothetical statement and then analyze your reaction. Here goes. "I believe Atkins is the best diet ever." You probably had one of the two following reactions:

- You're a lunatic. Atkins is the most unhealthy, unbalanced eating plan that ever existed.
- You're absolutely right! Atkins is the best thing that ever happened to me.

Which one is right? I'm going to go out on a limb and say neither reaction is *right*, per se. Both are somewhat right and somewhat wrong. Like so many things in life, many factors are involved.

If you had the first reaction then you're probably in the group who believes Atkins means eating bacon and eggs and steak for the rest of your born days. I honestly can't fault anyone for thinking that. The terms "low carb" and "Atkins" have been nearly synonymous for a very long time. Further, the term "low carb" is usually interpreted as "no carb." While it's true that strict carbohydrate restrictions are the hallmark of the Atkins induction phase, many people who find great success during this period are loath to give it up. To outsiders looking in, they see a majority of Atkins followers sticking to the induction phase forever. And that probably means eating bacon and eggs and steak all the time.

The primary criticism of Atkins is that it's harmful—harmful in two ways. First, a diet high in fat is a fast track to a heart attack. Second, the body needs carbohydrates to function. The body simply can't get all the nutrients it needs out of the limited foods allowed on the low (or no) carb plan. In short, the plan recommends everything that goes against conventional wisdom, and therefore must be bad.

I would be forced to agree with this too, if Atkins truly meant eating zero carbs for the rest of your life. But it doesn't. It's about *controlling* carbohydrates, not eliminating them. You begin with a very low carb intake to kick-start your body. You then re-introduce carbs into your diet, slowly and with great control, until you find the point at which they begin to cause damage. Eventually, you find a healthy, balanced diet which (surprise, surprise) can include cereal, bread, rice, nuts, fruits, vegetables, and everything else the mass media has told you is forbidden on Atkins. It disallows large quantities of high-glycemic foods and that's probably as it should be. As I said, no diet allows you to eat all the birthday cake you want. It doesn't dictate the exact number of carbohydrate grams you can have a day because that number is different for everyone. If you're a couch potato, the number will be pretty darn low. If you're a triathlete, it will be pretty darn high. No two "Atkins" diets will ever look the same, because no two people are the same.

If you had the second reaction, ("it's the best thing ever!") then you're probably one of those who has found great success on this plan at one time or another. If so, then I congratulate you. Hopefully you lost the weight you wanted to and kept it off. But *more* importantly, hopefully you did it correctly. If you got addicted to the large induction weight loss, you may have found it too irresistible to give up. But do be careful. The diet was *not* designed to work that way. You must eventually find your balance.

While this plan tends to get most of the credit (or blame) for all that is low carb dieting, it isn't the only one. In fact, it wasn't even the first. That distinction is generally bestowed upon two men, Dr. William Harvey and an undertaker named William Banting. The year was 1862.

Banting, like so many of us, began putting on weight in his thirties. He spent years and years trying to get control of it, but all in vain. No matter what he tried, he never made any headway into solving his problem. Banting, at five feet four inches tall, had reached 202 pounds by age 64. Along with the weight came other issues, particularly with sight and hearing. The latter problem ultimately brought him to Dr. Harvey, an ear, nose and throat specialist. Harvey was the first doctor Banting had seen who finally considered that there was a direct link between his health issues and his excess weight.

Harvey told Banting to eliminate six of his favorite (and as he thought them, innocent) foods: bread, butter, milk, sugar, beer, and potatoes. Alarmed at the time, Banting later wrote, "I had little left to live upon." Fortunately, Dr. Harvey provided him with ample dietary alternatives and he decided to take one more shot at solving his problem. The results were stunning. Within a very few days he found "immense benefit from it." Between August and December, he was down to 184 pounds. By the following August, just one year after he began, he reached 156 pounds. His vision and hearing improved. He suddenly found he could sleep through the night. He could actually bend over and tie his own shoes. He declared he hadn't felt that well in twenty-six years.

But it wasn't until after he'd achieved his goal that he did something truly incredible: he decided to write about it. He published a pamphlet covering both the diet and his own remarkable journey.* It's a fascinating read and full of all sorts of things we assume are modern inventions. My favorite: "I do not recommend every corpulent man to rush headlong into such a change of diet (certainly not), but to act advisedly and after full consultation with a physician."

The booklet was, by all accounts, the first ever best-seller

* Sheesh! What kind of guy would be crazy enough to think anyone would want to read about his dieting stories?

on dieting. By the time he wrote the fourth edition in 1869, it had already sold 63,000 copies and was available across the globe. He wasn't in it for the money either. In his own words:

> "Of all the parasites that affect humanity I do not know of, nor can I imagine, any more distressing than that of Obesity. [...] I am desirous of circulating my humble knowledge and experience for the benefit of other sufferers, with an earnest hope that it may lead to the same comfort and happiness I now feel under the extraordinary change."

About one hundred and thirty years later, I had wrapped up my own research on the topic. I was definitely intrigued by all that I had read. Apparently, this system wasn't as strange as it sounded. There was actually a method to the madness. The basic concept said if you restrict intake of the body's primary fuel source, the body has no choice but to fall back on burning its stores. In other words, stop eating donuts, and the donuts your body has been saving for the last ten years will finally get used. True, Atkins wasn't without controversy, but in my mind, the pros far outweighed the cons, and I was desperate for something—*anything*—to work.

So by early 2001, I was ready to go. Almost. I had just taken a new job in Austin, Texas which meant preparing for a big move and traveling back and forth for meetings. Life was a bit too chaotic to settle in with a new eating plan just yet. I also caught a tenacious cold, and wanted to wait a couple weeks until I was feeling well before my "full consultation with a physician."

When I finally saw my doctor, I wasn't sure what he'd say when I told him about the low-carb plan. I knew it was a divisive subject and didn't really want to get into a discussion about it, having already made up my mind. My fears were unfounded as he agreed that it could be a very useful tool for dropping excess tonnage. With that, my little project was a go.

That night I went grocery shopping. Let me tell you,

there's nothing quite like the unique rush of buying all new foods on the eve of a new feeding program. It's like buying paper, pencils, and Elmer's glue before the first day of school—nothing but good feelings over the promise of a brand new day.

I walked around the store like a kid in a candy shop. I was suddenly allowed—nay, *encouraged*—to buy all the things that were strictly forbidden on every other diet I'd ever tried. I can't say that I didn't feel a little naughty filling up my shopping cart with sausage, eggs, salami, cheese, pickles, pepperoni, bacon, heavy cream, nuts, and full-fat salad dressings. Although I'd done all the research and I understood the mechanics of what was about to happen, I still stared into that cart in disbelief. Overcoming decades of conventional wisdom overnight wasn't easy.

After I got home and put away the groceries, I set out to do a little cabinet cleansing. It was like a Mardi Gras party—my own private free-for-all before giving up all vices. I seized the opportunity to rid the pantry of all remaining soon-to-be-forbidden junk by shoving it down my carb hole. I remember little of the event, as I was loopy on the insulin rush. Hopefully I didn't flash anyone for beads.

The next morning I woke up in an absolutely thrilled mood. This part I remember quite clearly, because I'd never felt anything quite like it before—or since. The enthusiasm I experienced at the grocery store was now redoubled. I thought to myself, "Wow! This is it. Today is really the day." A large part of that was due to the fact that I'd made up my mind about this nearly six weeks earlier. So I had a *long* time to psych myself up for this. "The day has finally arrived!"

It was Thursday, February 15, 2001. I'd never started a diet on a Thursday before. It just naturally fell out that way, due to the doctor appointment being the day before. Besides, now that the Switch had been flipped on, the exact day of the week mattered little.

I bounded downstairs like a kid on Christmas morning

and cooked up two sausage patties and two eggs. Yum! What a great start. This *can't* be a diet, I thought to myself, still in disbelief. After breakfast, I packed up lunch and other food for the day and headed off to work. At the time, I worked in a small, three-room office with just a handful of other people. As I put my goods away in the fridge, a co-worker noticed the package of pepperoni slices in my hand.

"What's that?" He asked.

"Pepperoni," I replied.

"I see that. What's it for?"

"Just to snack on," I offered.

"Um, okay...," he said.

It was clear eating raw pepperoni as a snack was an alien concept. It was, of course—but unlike my perplexed office mates, I'd already had a fair amount time to warm up to the idea. Though it was the first inkling I had that this diet would likely require a lot of explanation. Keep in mind that 2001 was still before the low-carb craze hit, so explanations were in order.

The remainder of the day went well. The highlight was a big chicken Caesar salad for lunch—a meal that would soon become a staple of this plan. For those of you keeping score at home, the day's stats ended up like this:

	Grams	Calories	Percent
Fat	**144**	**1295**	**74%**
Saturated	58	518	30%
Polyunsaturated	24	220	13%
Monounsaturated	52	465	27%
Other/Unknown	10	92	5%
Protein	**99**	**396**	**23%**
Carbs	**19**	**55**	**3%**
Fiber	5	0	0%
Total	**262**	**1746**	**100%**

There are two remarkable things about this data. First, that is a *lot* of fat. Three quarters of the day's calories were from fat sources. Second, that's not a lot of calories. (Heck, I can down seventeen hundred calories in a single, nighttime snack attack.) In fact, that's one of the many criticisms of low carb programs. Critics say there's no magic about carbohydrate restriction. The typical mantra goes:

> "A calorie, is a calorie, is a calorie."
>
> "The sole reason low carb dieters lose weight is good, old-fashioned caloric reduction—just like every other diet."

I might be inclined to agree with this, if all I had to go on was the above chart. But as everyone knows, the *first* day of a diet *always* has the lowest number of calories. It only goes up from there. We'll explore this issue a bit more later on. For now, let's move on to Day Two.

I had an omelet the second morning, just to be different. Not that there was anything wrong with plain sausage and eggs; but an omelet feels a bit heartier. For lunch, I had a couple hot dogs and a salad. Pickles and cheese made good snacks during the day. I wrapped things up with a couple bratwursts. The caloric intake for the day: 2089. Fat was 77%, protein was 20%, and carbs were 3%.

The first two weeks of the program went very much like this. I had one odd day where I only ate 1200 calories, while on another day I took in 2200 calories. My daily carbohydrate intake ranged from eight to nineteen grams. In short, I was doing it. The strangest thing of all, I felt fine. In fact, I felt *better* than fine. This seemed like the most natural thing in the world. I didn't crave bread or potatoes or breakfast cereal. I craved *results*. After years and years of defeat, I had at last set my mind firmly on success and I would accept nothing less. That alone gave me the strength to reject anything that wasn't part of the plan.

Atkins and most other low-carb programs work by instigating a metabolic change in your body. By severely limiting carbohydrate intake, the body is forced into a metabolic stage called *ketosis*. This is the point where the liver has depleted its stores of glycogen but still somehow must provide the body with fuel. In order to fulfill these duties, it turns to fat for fuel. This is "fat burning" in its most literal sense. This is also the primary reason why a true low carb plan is not the same thing as just "cutting down on carbs." The entire point of all this is to get into ketosis. The point is to burn your donut storage. This is why cheating on this program is not the same as cheating on other diets.

While reading the Atkins book, one sentence above all others really hit home. He emphatically stated that if something "is not on your diet, you are to have absolutely none of it. Your 'just this one taste won't hurt' rationalization is the kiss of death." There are two reasons for this.

1. You have a problem. You eat too much. You wouldn't give a recovering alcoholic a drink and say, "Just this one taste won't hurt." By that same logic, *don't eat the damn Ding Dong.* You might be able to rationalize it mathematically, but we know rationale has nothing to do with dieting.

2. You're changing your body's metabolic functions. You have switched into burn mode. If you eat that Ding Dong your pancreas will yell, "Party time!" and it's all over. You will leave ketosis *instantaneously*. It can take several days to recover from one slip.

Now we have the full picture of what kept me going. I was completely fed up with myself. I wanted this to work more than anything. And to seal the deal, I had received a dire warning about the smallest amount of cheating being the kiss of death. For some people, this is too much. "The diet is too strict. The diet has no variety. The diet forbids cheating of any sort." Many would call this a recipe for disaster, and for a majority (including many I know personally) this indeed was their exact experience with Atkins. But no two people are alike. For me, this is *exactly* what I needed *exactly* when I needed it.

By the end of the first two weeks, I'd eaten over four pounds of fat and lost eleven pounds. The one thing I didn't do was exercise. I knew I *should* be exercising, but I really wanted to see what the dietary change was capable of accomplishing all on its own.

The next two weeks were much like the first two weeks. I was supposed to be out of the induction phase and starting to re-introduce carbohydrates into my diet. The only problem with that is I was hooked. Things were going so well on so many levels, I didn't want to risk messing that up: neither by cheating nor by following the prescribed plan. By the end of the first month, I was down fifteen pounds.

One of the best side effects of losing weight is being able to fit into new clothes. And "new" doesn't necessarily mean "new from the store." I'm sure for many other successful dieters, the chance to buy brand-new, smaller clothes from the store is the greatest payoff there is, exceeding even health benefits. I'm not that type. I'd be very surprised if I've personally (and voluntarily) shopped for new clothes more than twice in the last sixteen years.

No, for me, "new clothes" means just re-discovering the old ones. I head into the closet like an archaeologist on a dig, uncovering older and older artifacts the deeper I go. The trip to the back is like a trip through time. "Hey look, I wore these pants in sixth grade! I can—*grunt*—almost get into them again!"

So *my* new clothes are anything but. The best find for me is always a previously out-of-reach pair of jeans. There's no greater victory than adding a newly recovered pair to one's clothing arsenal. Unfortunately, they're typically in the worst shape possible. For one thing, they're old. For another, at the point where I finally gave up and stopped wearing them, they were already too small and showing signs of wear. In fact, they're probably still too small: my only real triumph is the fact that I can button them while standing up. But I take what I can get and off I go, wearing them proudly. "Hey, look everybody! Check out my *new* pants." More often than not, that happy feeling comes to a disheartening halt around a week later when I realize these new-yet-still-too-small jeans have worn clean through in the vicinity of the inside upper thighs.

"Damn!" I say to myself, examining the wreckage in the closet that evening. "Another perfectly good pair of jeans lost to chub rub."

On the occasions I am lucky enough to keep them for longer than a week, I then have to wrestle with the prospect of washing them. I try to put this off for as long as humanly possible, ignoring mustard and grease stains for far longer than is socially acceptable. Laura will sneak into the closet while I'm asleep, throw them in the washer, and replace them before I'm ever aware of what happened. The next day, in an attempt to put them on, I find I can only get them halfway up my tree trunks.

"Arrrrgh!"

Never wash a fat guy's jeans...

Still, I can't (or shouldn't) complain. These are all very minor issues to worry about given how well my overall diet program was going. The only other downside I can (or should?) complain about was my dietary incompatibility with the rest of the world. I never ate the same meals as the rest of my family or co-workers. I was the guy who threw out the cheeseburger buns and only ate the pizza toppings, but eventually everyone (including me) got used to it, and that's just the way I was.

There wasn't a great deal of variety in my diet either, but

I'm not the type of person who needs that. I felt no inclination to give in to temporary cravings (on the rare occasions even when I was tempted). I lived by the belief that *temptations are temporary but pizza is permanent.* I would ask myself something like, "What did you eat on April 17, 1995?" When I couldn't answer, I would then challenge myself, "Well, how about the 18th?" It was easy to realize that whatever I was feeling in the past was done and gone—gone beyond all recall. It helped me realize how temporary *right now* is and (more importantly) how pointless it would be to give into a temptation. Moreover, I was treating this like boot camp. What mattered to me wasn't the moment. What mattered was the future.

At restaurants, it was rather common to find nothing suitable to eat on the menu, thus causing me to fall back on the chicken Caesar salad. (I became quite the connoisseur over time.) Further, "suitable to eat" was not synonymous with "allowed on the diet." I am, as most everyone close to me knows, a very picky eater. I grew up on peanut butter and jelly sandwiches and very little else. For whatever reason, by nature or by nurture, I have a very limited palate. This used to bother me quite a bit, primarily for social reasons, but as I've grown older, I've learned to accept the fact that that's simply the way I am and it's never going to change.

I never could understand why foods others so obviously considered delicacies tasted so dreadful to me. By symmetry, others could never understand how on earth I could possibly prefer a 95¢ cheeseburger over a $95 caviar. The answer was abundantly clear to me: the cheeseburger tasted wonderful and the caviar tasted like banana slugs.

But picky eating shouldn't have been a problem at all, right? This *was*, of course, a low carb diet—with little or no variety. How could I possibly have any troubles being a picky eater? Oddly enough, I did. You might find this exceptionally strange, considering how well the low carb lifestyle suited me, but I don't actually like a wide range of meat products.

This comes as a shock to no one more than John.* A friend and co-worker, he is also the gracious host and proud sponsor of a quasi-annual event called Meat Fest. The basic premise is simple: buy and cook three hundred pounds of meat and have a few friends over to eat it. It's a monumental effort, but he's rarely happier than when he's cooking food and feeding friends. Fortunately, for me, Mr. Picky, Meat Fest has plenty of hamburgers, sausages, turkey and other things I very much like to eat. However, I suppose I always run the risk of showing up some year and it's nothing but roast beef.

It's really quite tragic, considering meat is the hallmark of the low carb diet, but it's the truth. Some types of meat I'll eat if presented with them (but would never buy or seek out on my own). Other types I just don't care for at all. Consider this recent instant messaging chat:

Steph:	What should I make for dinner tonight? Last night was pot roast.
Me:	I don't much like pot roast, so I'm not sorry I missed that.
Steph:	ohhhhhh that's right, you don't like mushrooms
Me:	mushrooms? I said I don't like pot roast.
Steph:	well my pot roast always has cream of mushroom soup on it.
Me:	It also has pot roast in it, which I don't like.
Steph:	my pot roast is tender AND moist.
Me:	it's tender and moist AND pot roast.

So yeah, it's that bad sometimes. I'll venture to guess that this bit of info probably gives you a glimpse of how a typical

* Not his real name. Oh, who am I kidding? Of *course* it's his name. How can you give a pseudonym to someone named John?

restaurant outing might turn out.

"There's a nice leg of lamb here on the menu," my ever-helpful dinner companions point out. "That's meat! You can eat that."

"Sorry, but I *can't* eat that," is my apologetic reply.

"What about the liver?" they continue, determined to help me out on my bizarre diet.

"Nope, sorry again," I return.

"Well how about the..."

"I think I'll just get the chicken Caesar salad."

It's a sad state but I offer no more apologies. I've accepted my fate. Just remember, if we ever meet and you decide to treat me to a fancy dinner, just spring for a Happy Meal. You'll save a lot of money and we'll both be much happier.

About the only thing worse than serving me something I don't like is serving me something I *do* like, but can't have. It was far more common for friends to unhelpfully persuade me to order a strictly *verboten* menu item.

"Oh, come on!" they would beg, in a doomed attempt to encourage me. "Just get a plate of pasta. You deserve it! One meal won't kill you."

"Yes it will," was my standard-issue reply.

They didn't understand the kiss of death. They couldn't realize what was at stake. But I knew. For me, the salad—even if for the seventy-third time—was the best option.

The weight loss continued. In my third month, I passed a very important milestone. On May 26, 2001, I stepped on the scale and saw 192. While that doesn't seem like a remarkable number at face value, it's where I passed the "it doesn't get any better than this" point from way back on page 41. Wow. It only took eight years, four hundred and seventy-two Day Ones, a thousand miles of walking, one marathon, and a miracle diet, but I did it.

The positive effects were rubbing off on those around me too. Even John began to think there was something about this "excessive carbohydrate" problem. He decided to do nothing more than give up Romulan noodles (as we liked to call them) and switch to diet sodas. He began to lose weight immediately. Another guy we worked with, Dustin,* started his own program. Was this due to me? Of course not. But he did end up dropping nearly one hundred pounds, and that alone is worth mentioning here. Like me, he's still at it today. Some of us never learn.

Eventually, my rate of weight loss slowed as expected. The week-to-week losses weren't as dramatic as they'd been at the beginning. I gradually introduced more calories and carbs into the mix, mostly through the form of mixed nuts or cashew pieces. The summer passed, and I kept at it, right on through fall. For the first time in my entire life, I didn't eat a single piece of candy at Halloween. This in itself was extraordinary, and an obvious testament that I had fundamentally changed my behavior.

The thing is, I fell into the trap of thinking the diet had done all this for me. What else could explain it? I'd tried and failed so many other things. It was obvious that the only way I could be sticking to the plan so well was because the diet had somehow bestowed the power of tenacity upon me. It was a medical miracle. I now know that wasn't the case at all, but at the time, it sure felt like it.

One evening in early November, we were at work late. (Being your typical start-up, this was hardly an unusual occurrence.) We were hungry and decided to go to Taco Bell for some grub. As I stood in line, I debated my choices, but ended up getting real tacos with real tortillas.† They were of the corn variety,

---

* His real name. There's nothing innocent about Dustin to protect.

† Yes, yes. I know Taco Bell isn't known for *real* tacos. I just meant "real" in the sense that they weren't special diet tacos (and they weren't a chicken Caesar salad).

so not as bad (carb-wise) as flour tortillas, but still more than I was used to. This was a real test. The *kiss of death* mantra still rang in my head. But I figured, *oh, what the heck.* One or two tacos can't kill me, right?

Physically, no. The tacos did not kill me. But it definitely took me one rung down the ladder, psychologically speaking. Looking back, I think this innocent event created a tiny crack in the windshield. It was nothing to worry about at the time, but it did set in motion far-reaching events. The butterfly had flapped its wings.

Anyway, we'll get to that mess soon enough. For now, let's see how the whole year went. Here's the happy chart:

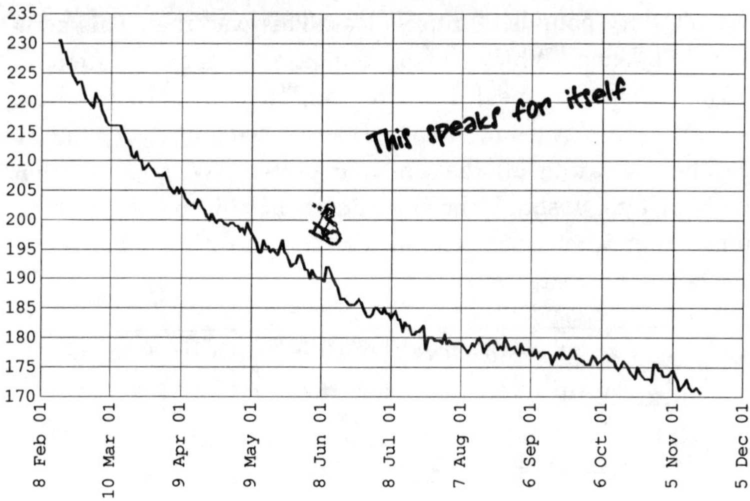

Total loss? Sixty pounds.

Total time? Two hundred and seventy six days.

Total success? I do believe so.

I don't care what anyone else says, *that* is an accomplishment. I mean, *wow*, look at that. I even made it down to 170 pounds again—something I truly believed was *impossible.* I'd long ago given up on that pipe dream, instead downshifting to the vain hope I could someday break back into Onederland.

Nothing else I tried seemed to stick until I suddenly got the bright idea to quit eating potato chips. Nine months later—*bam!*—all better now. Consider all those earlier attempts of mine. I walked a thousand miles and didn't lose anywhere near that much weight (even given twice the calendar time). I tried lifting weights and got nothing out of it. Why, I even breathed funny for two weeks. Still nothing. But this? I didn't exercise once. I didn't lift a finger. I just changed my diet. I still ate a whole bunch of calories every day, but because they weren't high-energy calories, my body was forced to use up the bulk of its fat storage.

Yes, it really was fat loss. To the various low carb detractors out there, this wasn't sixty pounds of water weight. This wasn't sixty pounds of muscle loss. This was real. This actually happened. Which means the last, obvious question is, "What about my health?" After all, there's more to losing weight than just losing weight. Doing it too quickly isn't good. Neither is eating all that fat and protein. With a diet that high in fats, I should be near-death at this point. Surprisingly, that wasn't the case at all. The following table shows the before and after results:

	Before	After	Normal
Cholesterol	165	159	< 200
Triglycerides	209	85	< 150
Blood Sugar	106	90s	70 to 100

My cholesterol went down slightly, but since it was well in the normal range before beginning (which still amazes me) this isn't that dramatic. My HDL and LDL levels (also normal at the start) both moved further in the right direction. My blood sugar dropped below one hundred, but I don't know the exact number because I can't find my notes from six years ago. "Why don't you just call the doctor and get the results?" Well, I tried that, but she seems to have vanished off the face of the planet. I can only assume she won the lotto, changed her name, and moved to a country without internet access.

Anyway, the most dramatic change was that of my triglyceride counts. High triglyceride levels can increase the risk of atherosclerosis. They are elevated through a lack of exercise, irregular eating patterns, diets high in saturated fats and sugars, and so on. (In other words, everything that described me before starting.) They are brought under control through exercise and a diet low in saturated fats. Ironic, then, that I lowered mine by *not* exercising and eating *more* saturated fats. What gives? Am I some kind of mutant? Not quite. You might be surprised to discover that the low carbohydrate diet was not created as a weight loss solution. It was designed to treat patients with serious health problems (in particular, heart disease and diabetes). Weight loss was just an unintended side effect of fixing the body's innards.

So we seem to have a paradox. If high fat diets were bad, and known to cause heart problems, why on earth would doctors purposefully put patients with heart disease on a high fat diet? Even stranger, why did these diets work, given what we know about the high fat diet? The answer should be obvious at this point. It's the carbohydrates. But wait a minute. Diets high in carbohydrates can't be bad. Lots of people have lost lots of weight on high carb diets. This doesn't make sense.

It *can* be confusing at face value but I think this stems from our natural tendency to over-simplify things. Traditional studies that demonstrated the dangers of high fat diets used subjects also eating high levels of carbohydrates. When the fat was reduced, the subjects fared better. The obvious conclusion? Fat must be bad. What these studies apparently overlooked was testing the *other* direction. That is, reduce the carbs, leave the fat, and *then* see what happens. It took a long while before anyone did that. It's almost as if "fat is bad" were a foregone conclusion. Hmmm...

But enough pseudo-scientific nonsense. The important thing right now is *me*. Before moving on to the next chapter, let's go over my astonishing results once again. ☺ It's even more impressive when you look at the last graph plotted alongside the entire dataset. This chart represents everything from my starting point in May 1990 until November 18, 2001.

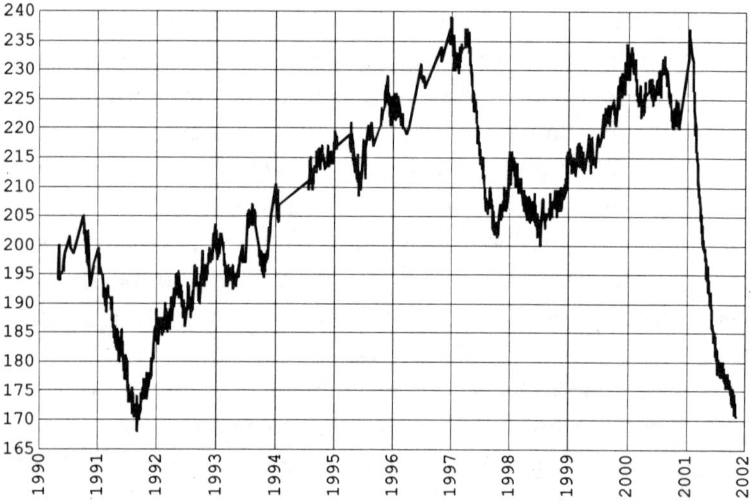

And he lived happily ever after.

As I look back on this today, even after years have passed, I still gaze at it in disbelief. I apologize for continuing to gush over these results, but I'd simply never experienced anything like it before. I don't know that I ever will again. You see, as terrible as it sounds, a series of unfortunate events is about to transpire. If you're wondering what could possibly happen, just look at the date again.

It's November 18.

Oh no.

Chapter 18

The Pancakes of Death

Living in Austin meant we were now almost a thousand miles from the nearest relatives. For this reason, we decided to forego the traditional Thanksgiving activities and take advantage of the long weekend. Our first mini vacation was spent in South Padre Island, Texas.

Given how well the previous nine months had gone coupled with how happy I was about my accomplishment added to how good I felt about myself only meant one thing: it was high time to put a stop to all that.

And the worst part? It was a completely conscious decision. I wasn't suckered into it. My atomic subcomponents didn't decide to fall off the wagon without consulting me. No, it was all my doing. I think after nine months, I might have gotten a bit cocky. Perhaps this "kiss of death" thing was just a load of nonsense. After all, what could possibly happen in one weekend? I clearly had the tools at my disposal to take care of anything. After all, I'd just lost sixty pounds, without any effort at all. Even if I did gain a couple pounds over the weekend, what's the worst that could happen? I'll just lose them again right away. No problem.

The trip began well. Although the car was filled with road snacks, I stuck to my normal eating plan. I didn't stray on the trip down or the first night either. You might think this was still out of sheer willpower and the desire to advance my goals even further. In truth, I simply didn't want to spoil my long-planned "reward."

The reward is an evil facet of every diet. "I've done good! I *deserve* this!" you tell yourself. Well let me tell you, nothing good has ever come from that kind of rationale. You work and work and work only to reward yourself with near-certain destruction. It's like spending a month building the perfect birdhouse with your borrowed tools, then setting it on fire to celebrate your accomplishment. But as I've said already, when has rational thinking ever come into play when it comes to eating?

The next morning we went downstairs to the hotel restaurant for breakfast. I didn't need to look at the menu. I knew exactly what I wanted: *pancakes*. Pancakes and butter and syrup. That's right. Daddy's been good all year and wants a little sugar. I've done good. I *deserve* this.

Many restaurants claim they serve so-called homemade pancakes. Well, I've made pancakes at home before and they're nothing like the manhole covers that most restaurants routinely produce. Mine are smallish, thin, and can actually be consumed in a few bites. Restaurants, on the other hand, delight in creating pancakes so large that they could be used as floatation devices in the unlikely event of a water landing. The wait staff delivers them to your table with a forklift. One alone would be more than enough for a meal, but for some reason they think you need three or four of them. "Here you go, sir! The ambulance is waiting just outside if you need it."

But I didn't care about any of that. I settled into my spot, anxious for my hard-earned reward. Everyone at the table stared at me with a sort of "are you really going to do this?" look. I'd been so militant for so long about the low carb program that this seemed unthinkable. This wasn't like me.

But I didn't care about any of that. Most of the people I met during 2001 only knew me as "the low carb guy." As far as they knew, I'd been doing it my entire life. It's just who I was. I stuck to it. I never fell off the wagon. Nothing got in my way. I lost sixty pounds.

But I didn't care about any of that. This was, after all, just one meal. Nine months of hard labor was not going to be adversely affected by one dang plate of pancakes.

The golden brown stack arrived with the required pancake accessories: whipped butter and hot syrup.* The trick is to place layers of butter between the pancakes and ensure that not a square centimeter of pancake surface area is left untouched by the syrup. If you hit a dry spot, then by all means get it soaked in maplely goodness before continuing. Otherwise you're just going through the motions.

The pancakes were everything I'd hoped they'd be. The long wait was definitely worth it. Each bite was a little bit of hot, griddled ecstasy. I honestly don't remember if I actually finished them all or not, but it didn't matter, for the wheels were set in motion.

When you go a long time with stable blood sugar levels, your body essentially operates the way it was designed. The sudden assault of monosaccharides on my body and the subsequent insulin rush gave new meaning to the term sugar high. I felt lightheaded, somewhat loopy, and rather good—in a not-so-good sort of way. I began to understand how this really could be considered a toxin, illegal drug, or both.

We conducted normal beach-related, vacation-like activities for the next several hours until it was time for our long-awaited Thanksgiving dinner. I had three primary objectives for this meal:

---

* Wouldn't *Pancake Accessories* be a great band name? For that matter, both *Whipped Butter* and *Hot Syrup* would work too. I think coming up with band names is more fun than playing in one.

Objective #1: **Mashed Potatoes**. Done right, the mashed potato is nothing short of whipped heaven. The trick is to make them very fluffy, pile them up in a big bowl like a volcano, and top them with enough butter that it pours down the sides like lava.

Objective #2: **Stuffing**. No Turkey Day meal would be complete without stuffing drenched in gravy. Just be sure to cook it *in the bird* just as we've done for the last four hundred years. Bacteria shmacteria. It's only once a year.

Objective #3: **Pumpkin Pie**. Last, but certainly not least, is the pie. If I could, I'd whip it up fluffy, pile it up in a big bowl like a volcano, and top it with enough whipped cream that it pours down the sides like lava.

We searched the island up and down for a buffet and found one in a hotel. For just $22.50 per person, they offered All You Can Eat mashed potatoes, stuffing, and pumpkin pie. There might have been other offerings, such as pickles and maybe turkey, but I wasn't really paying attention.

The good news is we had plenty to go around. But this story is not without bad news. First, mashed potatoes are notoriously difficult to keep warm. Heat escapes from potatoes faster than Houdini from handcuffs. If I'd had my way, I would have gone right into the kitchen itself and scooped them into my mouth straight from the pot. But I didn't need another potato-related restraining order, so I opted to serve myself from the buffet table. They were only mildly warm and regrettably lava-free. The stuffing was passable. Not terrific, and certainly nothing I'd write a book about. And the pie? Guess what. There *was* no pumpkin pie! It was worse than spending weeks driving to Wally World and finding it closed. The moose out front should have told us. The months and months of carbohydrate denial ended in pumpkinless tragedy.

The real tragedy, however, had not yet begun. The next day, with my spree behind me, I assumed I would get right back on the program. My fling was over, so I should have been able to continue on my way as if nothing had ever happened.

But something happened all right. My body, suddenly remembering, "Ah, so *that's* what life used to be like!" decided it wanted more—*lots* more. My brain sent out bulletins to every corner of the body, calling for action. "Whatever it takes, boys! Just get some more of that stuff down here!"

To make a long and painful story short and painful, I ended up gaining seven pounds between November 22 and November 26, 2001. That's right. In just five short days, I gained seven pounds (or about one pound every eighteen hours). Someone once told me, "If you're going to step over the line, you might as well jump." I definitely jumped. I should probably call Guinness.

That first morning back home, my mind reeled as I nervously approached the scale to fully assess the damage. How bad would it be? How bad *could* it be? I knew that I, um, strayed a little over the holiday but never expected a seven-pound gain. When I peered down and saw 179.5 at my feet, my jaw dropped. This was almost worse than any number starting with a two. On that day, I wrote:

> Yowza! Went off the wagon and look what happened! I guess I kind of enjoyed it, but mostly I didn't. I'm VERY anxious to get back on the program.

"Mostly didn't enjoy it?" What could I possibly mean by that? Well, I'll tell you. The whole trip was a nightmare. I was an automaton again—cursing every bite and utterly helpless to stop it. It was like being a marionette, with an evil, invisible puppeteer overhead mercilessly and relentlessly bringing hand to mouth.

I never realized the *kiss of death* meant *just that.* This wasn't just about pausing the weight loss, or coming out of ketosis, or gaining a couple pounds back. Giving the body back what it so desperately craved was doom.

And the sad part is I didn't even have to do it. I *wanted* to do it. The whole sordid affair was premeditated, for crying out loud. I did it on purpose.

I was somehow able to take the next couple weeks and work my way back down to 173. But it stopped right there. It just wasn't going to get any better than that.

Not for a long, long time.

Chapter 19

Flailing

When I first embarked on the low carb lifestyle, I remember wishing that I had as many grocery store options as the low fat dieters did. It seemed unfair that when low fat diets swept the nation, the shelves filled with low fat and fat free offerings. Never mind that most of them were horrible products, just barely cracking the FDA's definition of "food." At least dieters had a choice.

That all changed when the low carb craze hit. Just as I was falling off my perfect diet, the rest of the world had hit critical mass. That's the point where the food industry sees a fast buck to be made and floods the market to meet the demands of the latest trend.

At first, I was somewhat dismayed at the timing. "Why didn't this hit in 2001, when I needed it?" Then my mood shifted, and I was pleasantly pleased by the attention "my" diet was getting. In some ways, I felt it had validated what I'd done. But those feelings were short-lived. Soon the craze went through the roof. Some manufacturers made low-carb alternatives to their regular products. Others who already offered low-carb products suddenly shouted it from the rooftops.

Products you'd never think of as "low carb" were suddenly low in carbs. I remember gazing dumbfounded at beer commercials showing men and women alike with six-pack abs, somehow implying that the more six packs of beer you drank, the thinner you'd be. Stranger still was the introduction of low carb soft drinks. Never mind that *no* carb soft drinks had already been in existence for fifty years. New *low* carb soft drinks were now something new. I'm not sure if going from forty to twenty grams of carbohydrates was ever going to solve anything in the long run, but if it moves products off the shelves, that's all that matters. The last straw for me was low carb breakfast cereal. That's right. Someone invented low carb carbs. Crazy.

Naturally, whenever a craze hits, nutritionists come out of the woodwork to denounce said craze. Newspapers, magazines, morning shows, and talk shows all trot out the experts to tell us how stupid we are for blindly following the crowd. The attacks on low carb were predictable. "It's too high in fat! Studies show that high fat diets lead to instant death." Trouble is, they were quoting all those studies that showed how diets high in fat *and* high in carbs affected the body. The body reacts completely differently to diets high in fat and low in carbs.

I will agree with them on one point. Many people *were* blindly attempting a low carb diet without any clear idea what they were doing. I imagine more than one person out there ate three bowls of low carb cereal for breakfast, drank eight low carb sodas during the day, and downed two low carb beers at night. I guess I can't blame them for wanting to set the record straight.

For better or worse, I missed the whole craze. I made a few half-hearted attempts again at living la vida low carb, but nothing stuck. The fad passed me by and I began to look for other things to whip me back into shape.

In August 2002, I was back in Chicago on a family visit.

One or both of my sisters had stumbled across some kind of bodybuilding makeover program. They eagerly trotted out the book and we poured over the stunning "before and after" photographs. They were amazing. People went from looking like—well, from looking like me to looking like the Incredible Hulk, except not as green.

"What's the deal with this?" I asked them.

"It's basically bodybuilding. You just work out like a madman for twelve weeks, and you end up like this."

"Really? Twelve weeks? Look at these people!" I couldn't believe it was possible.

This was, as you may have already guessed, the Body for Life program. Both Beth and Jenn seemed interested in it, and after a short amount of pondering, I found myself wanting to give it a shot too. I began to have wild fantasies about looking like all the guys shown in those after photos. "You could look like that before Thanksgiving!" I told myself, half believing it.

As soon as I returned from my trip, I hit my first real hurdle: getting the garage cleaned up. When we moved from Des Moines to Austin, we left more than cold winters behind us. We left basements. This meant that everything that *used* to be in our cluttered basement was now in our cluttered garage. I began to realize I would probably lose ten pounds just trying to set up a workout area.

Eventually the deed was done. A small area was cleared just enough to fit an old, secondhand workout bench with some assorted free weights. It felt good to be moving forward again. I celebrated my accomplishment with another big plate of pancakes.

Monday, August 26, 2002 dawned. It was hard to believe it was time for yet another Day One. I woke up about an hour earlier than usual—not hard considering how anxious I was to begin the new workout program. (You know, sometimes I wish every day could be a Day One. They're the best.) After getting out of bed, I checked my weight*, threw on some sweats, walked right past the pancakes, and into the dimly lit, and altogether uninviting garage. The weights sat there, cold and hard, but I was ready for 'em.

I thought I would start out slow. It didn't make sense to jump right into the heavy stuff and risk bodily injury. I carefully slid 150 pounds of weights onto each end of the weight bar and did about thirty bench press reps.

NOT.

Actually, I started out with an empty bar, which was more than enough weight for this mushy spud. I moved between various presses, curls, and leg lifts. The session lasted all of about forty-five minutes. By the time I was done, the rest of the house was awake. I made my way to the kitchen, about as flexible as the Tin Man rusted shut in the woods.

"How'd the first workout go?" Laura asked.

"*Oil can...*" I replied slowly through locked teeth.

I was stiff and sore, that's for sure. I don't know how the body is able to keep masses of muscles out of everyday use for so long. At least it has the ability to call on them when needed.

The plan called for alternating days of weightlifting vs. aerobic activity. On Day Two, I headed out for a brisk walk. This was much better! Walking was something I was good at and even remembered how to do.

The next four days continued to alternate between the two workouts. The seventh day, by contrast, was a designated free day. On this day, you don't have to exercise and can eat anything you want. The idea is simple: your body needs rest. It also helps to mix it up a little, so your body doesn't settle into a pattern. Lastly, it provides a good psychological break. It can be *very* daunting (if not downright discouraging) to think you have to eat right and exercise seven days a week for the rest of your life with nary a break.

---

* 186 pounds. Not too bad, actually. I really was able to hold things together for most of 2002.

Body for Life isn't the only program that allows one free day a week. Me? I treat this day off differently. I don't take a day off. Sure, it looks great on paper. Mathematically, there's no evidence it should do any long-term damage. However, in my case, it's just not a good thing at all. If I've spent an entire week eating well and working out then the *last* thing I need is an excuse to throw it all away. I do that fine on my own without any external encouragement. I've known people who've done diets with free days and I've heard them talk about how much they were looking forward to eating for twelve hours straight. "It's okay! The diet says it's okay!"

Talk about the kiss of death.

Aside from knowing I'd fall off the wagon and never get back on, in the back of my mind lived the thought of the competition. I signed up for the challenge. I was going to take these twelve weeks seriously and I *knew*, judging from the spectacular before and after photos, that *none* of these people turned every seventh day into a twelve hour feed fest. No, they were definitely going above and beyond the call of duty.

The second week began, and I stuck to it. The third and fourth weeks passed, and I was still at it. By now, I was actually putting weights on the bars, working harder reps, walking more quickly, and (much to my surprise) I was seeing some real results. My arms and shoulders weren't just featureless mounds of flesh anymore. There was actual muscle definition. "Wow," I thought. "This might just actually work."

There were, as you might expect, days where I didn't feel like getting up at all. But as I lay in my unrelentingly comfy bed, all I could think of were the previous years' winners. A little voice in my head whispered, "Winners don't stay in bed," and up I'd get. As each day rolled by, I felt stronger and stronger. There was one day in particular I remember picking up my six-year daughter and thinking she'd lost twenty pounds. I didn't struggle to lift her off the ground. Amazing.

And he lived happily ever after.

At least you think he should have. For some reason, even though I kept up with the workouts, I started eating more. The struggle between food and exercise became an issue once again. There's this small part of you that thinks it's perfectly fine to eat more just because of the exercising. What's easy to forget is that calories are taken in *far* easier than they're expended—even on an intense program. "I'm working out! Pass me those potatoes again." "Pizza? It's all right. I walked a mile this morning. I'll have another slice or two (or six)."

By the end of the eleventh week, I was about as fit and strong as ever, but now weighed 187. Yeah, yeah. I've heard it already. Muscle weighs more than fat. Still, there was no doubt I was already over-eating again. The exercising just kept it at bay for a while. It didn't solve anything.

I also didn't look any better, from a bodybuilding point of view. I peaked around the sixth week, and that was about that. Looking at my own dismal results, I seriously began to doubt that any of those people actually accomplished their goals in just three months, as the photos imply.

And right on cue, the twelve-week program ended right at Thanksgiving. I quit working out, kept right on eating, and by January 1, 2003 was back above 190.

The next year can probably be best summed up by these actual entries taken straight from my weight spreadsheet:

> January 1, 2003: New Day One: Goal for 2003 is to lose 21 pounds and 4 inches off the waist.
>
> February 15: Two Year Anniversary of Low-Carb. [Oh, man! If only I'd just *stuck to it!* What was I thinking? Pancakes? Sheesh!]
>
> March 24: Bad weekend. I think I'll call this a new Day One.
>
> April 14: So much for that last Day One.

May 5: Yes, another day one. But I'm serious this time!

June 16: Ack! Time for YADO [yet another day one]

June 23: No, TODAY is Day One

June 30: No, TODAY is Day One. Really, I mean it.

And on and on it went. I'll spare you (and me) the remainder of the year. You can see these are clearly the ramblings of an insane human being. There are no rational thought processes at work here. I kept thinking to myself, *you can do this*. But that evidently wasn't the case at all.

Things really hit home on January 6, 2004 as I crossed back over into the 200s. This was a hard one. After the 2001 miracle, I *swore* I'd never go back into the 200s. I was so sure and so confident that I had all the tools in the world to help me that I'd never, ever get that bad again. Yeah, maybe a few pounds here or there—maybe ten or fifteen tops in my wildest nightmares. But I was sure I'd always be able to stop it any time I wanted. Any damn time at all.

Then *wham!* There I was back where I said I'd never, ever be. The last time my weight began with "2" was April 26, 2001. In less than three years, I'd found my way back.

It sure got me motivated. Unfortunately, the motivation never translated into results. The year was peppered with dietlets. I managed to get back down to about 195 a few times along the way, but nothing was sticking.

Also, for the first time ever, I would cheat at the drop of a hat. It was never so easy.

"Want a slice of pizza?" someone would ask me.

"No," I'd reply firmly and with pride. "I'm on a diet!"

"Are you sure? It's yummy."

"Okay!"

This wasn't like me. It wasn't like me at all. But I didn't know what to do about it. Not at all. I had no plan, no tools, no help, and no hope.

I did conduct one interesting science experiment during this period. At least the premise was interesting. The actual results were pointless. The idea was to demonstrate calorie theory. Specifically, to show that an excess of 3,500 calories would make me gain a pound and that a deficit of 3,500 calories would make me lose a pound.

To do this, I first had to establish a baseline: the caloric intake required to neither gain nor lose weight. Since I was in a hurry, I just got a guesstimate from some online calculator, based on my weight, gender, and height. I then carefully constructed a meal plan that would be exactly 500 calories over that figure. If I could do that for two weeks, I would gain exactly two pounds. (Yes, it was my first-ever diet designed to gain weight.) Once I met that goal, I would back off to the base intake for two weeks, to demonstrate that no weight would be lost. Finally, I would eat 500 fewer calories for two weeks and see if I would lose two pounds.

To eliminate as many external factors as possible, I kept my exercising at the exact same levels every day (i.e., none). I also ate the exact same thing every day at the same time every day. The diet generally followed the Food Pyramid—not because it was the be-all, end-all of diet plans, but primarily due to its being a generally accepted middle-of-the-road solution. Additionally, I imposed the following rules on myself:

- Keep sodium below three grams per day.
- No caffeine or alcohol.
- No artificial sweeteners.
- No fake food (*especially* "fat free" crud).
- Add vitamin supplements.
- Drink at least sixty-four ounces of water each day.
- Six meals a day.

Not a bad plan overall, actually. I should try something like this again. Well, except for maybe the water part. I'm not sure what it is about requiring a tall glass of water every hour. The theory goes that it keeps your innards properly lubed up and cleaned out. For me, the negatives far outweigh the positives. In fact, I nearly got fired one week for spending six hours a day peeing. What's the point?

Anyway, Day One of the Great Caloric Experiment was Monday, July 19, 2004. My initial weigh-in was 212 pounds. The idea was to eat 3,000 calories, which I found *incredibly difficult* to do given the above constraints. When you're down to just eating grains, fruits, and veggies, packing on the pounds is a feat in and of itself. The first day was a disaster. I missed my planned fifth and six meals. Then, before going to bed hungry, I fixed a package of Ramen noodles.* Even so, I only ate 1,750 calories for the day and the next morning I weighed in at 209.5.

I can't get a break, can I? The one time I design a diet to gain weight, I lose two and a half pounds overnight. The next day didn't go any better, nor the next. As it turns out, there was no way I could overeat once I'd eliminated all the junk. So I decided to switch gears. I thought, "I'll just pick the amount of food I *can* eat, and then stick to that."

And so I did. I ate the exact same thing every day until about the second week of September. At that point I found myself weighing in at 197.5—a loss of 14.5 pounds in less than eight weeks.

And he lived happily ever after.

The normal (that is to say, *sane*) person would use these results as a positive, motivating factor in his life and keep right at it—but not me. I decided to add one free meal per week into the program. At first, I justified it in the name of science. Well, no, at *first*, I did it because after almost seven weeks, I just wanted something different to eat. It was Labor Day weekend and we decided to spend a couple of days painting. I was hot, tired, and worn out after a full day of applying

---

* This is a very great food product, by the way. I don't care *what* Stephanie says about them.

masking tape, painting walls, and cleaning brushes. We ordered Chinese food, and I got one of my all-time favorites, sesame chicken.

Wow. It was *good*. It was really, *really* good. It struck me immediately that this was probably how life was *supposed* to work. My thoughts strayed back to prehistoric peoples surviving on the same food day in and day out—and then about how they might have felt at a feast celebrating a hunt. The food alone didn't make it special. The infrequency of the event was every bit as important. One *had* to appreciate it. There was no way it could be otherwise. Now return to modern times. What has happened to the feast? Oh, we still have them. In fact, most of us have three or more of them a day. Our everyday meals—from softball-sized muffins to super-sized burger baskets—have become feasts compared to the everyday meals of the past. We feast and we feast and we feast. We feast on Who-pudding and rare Who-roast beast. Then, when a *really* special occasion comes along, we double or triple our intake. It's all quite sad, actually.

But anyway, there I was, enjoying my first real meal in seven weeks. When it ended, I was stuffed, but I wanted more. Not right then and there, but sometime soon. That's when it hit me: why *not* just eat one free meal a week? I could certainly lose weight the other 167 hours of the week—yet give myself something special to look forward to each weekend. It was the perfect plan.

And miraculously, I stuck to it. I was good all week and on Friday morning, I weighed in at 197.5. That same evening, the pizza showed up. I had a slice or two (or six) and reflected once again on the awesome specialness of eating like this.

Saturday morning dawned; time to pay the piper. I got up, went through the usual routine, and hopped on the scale.

"*What the bleep?!*" I exclaimed to my toes.

The scale read 195.5—down *two pounds* from the previous morning. Holy pepperoni, Batman! Had I actually discovered the mythical Pizza Diet?

The short answer is, "no," because on the next morning I'd *gained* three pounds. Damn! So much for that. Oddly enough, my weigh-ins for the following Friday, Saturday, and Sunday followed the same pattern: 196.5, 195.5, and 198.5.

And that's about as good as it was going to get. I still (mostly) kept to the plan but my one free meal a week was suddenly happening more than once a week. The last vestige of the original plan died on October 16, when I drank my first soda pop. And it was really, *really* good after going three months without. I should try that more often to maintain my appreciation levels. (Well, on second thought, naaah.)

One week later, it was over for good. I ate pounds of Halloween candy and by November first, I was back up to 204. And only two months after that, I was back up to 224.

Way to go, moron. Brilliant—just brilliant.

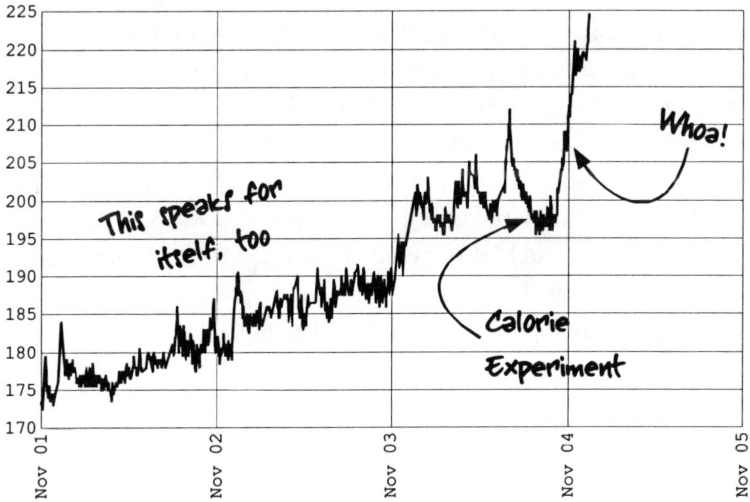

As you've no doubt guessed, I resumed dieting January 2005. I decided *this was it.* I had finally had enough. I decided to give the low-carb thing another serious go. After all, this plan worked like a miracle before, so it *had* to work again, right? There was only one trick as I saw it: I had to make sure I was truly serious about it. The Switch had to be on.

Before starting, though, I simply had to get myself some chicken planks from Long John Silvers; chicken planks with fries, hush puppies, and extra fries for slaw. Oh, and a small pile of those crumbly things too. [Insert Homer Simpson drooling sound here.] Boy, if I ever had to add a fifth food group to my ideal diet, it would definitely be chicken planks. Our feeble language has no words to describe them and their deep-fried breaded goodness. And there's definitely no explaining them at all to the unbeliever.

So with my last meal behind me, and the Switch hopefully in the "on" position, I began this latest diet attempt on my birthday. (The first and last time I've ever done *that*.)

By all appearances, the Switch was indeed on. I lost ten pounds in the first three weeks. The next week went well. I lost two more pounds but after that, something didn't feel right. I couldn't put my finger on it, but it's painfully obvious to me now what happened. The Switch never really was on. I didn't notice it back then, but all the signs were all there: the cravings, the temptations, and the extraordinary ease with which I would rationalize cheating. If I donated blood, I'd eat a fistful of cookies. If we were at a movie, I'd eat popcorn. If I attended a birthday party, I'd have cake.

This was in such stark contrast to the 2001 venture that it was almost as if I were a different person. In fact, sometimes I actually felt like two different people:

Sméagol: Oh no! Look! A box of Cheez-Its.

Gollum: Cheez-Its? Cheez-Its! We wants them! Yesss!

Sméagol: No! I hates them. They makes both of us crazy.

Gollum: No, not crazy. They makes us big and strong. We wants them! And we hates them what takes them from us! Thief Baggins stole our box a long time ago—*gollum, gollum.*

Sméagol: No! No crackerses! I want fishes instead. Nice, low-carb fishes!

In spite of my struggles, I never went *completely* off the wagon. But fundamentally, I knew things just weren't right. I should have read the signs when I found myself fixing low carb shakes for breakfast with chocolate chip mint ice cream.

Here's a side-by-side comparison of my 2001 low carb diet with the 2005 attempt, running from Day 1 to Day 180.

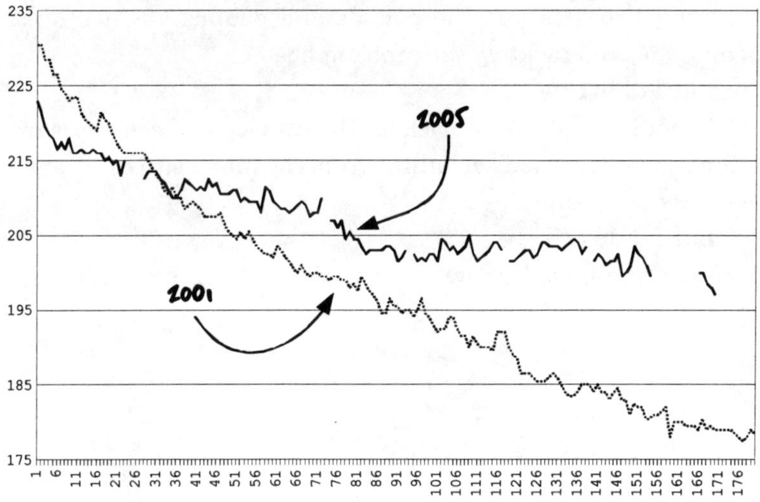

My last weigh-in of the year was 205.5, putting me down about nineteen pounds for the year. On the surface, this looks good. I mean, who would complain about losing nearly twenty pounds in a year? However, let's re-examine that in light of the following two bullet points:

- This was nothing compared to 2001. Granted, I shouldn't come to expect to lose sixty pounds in nine months every time I try a program. But this was *supposed* to be the *same dang program*. It was dreadfully disappointing.

- Nearly *half* of the year's loss was regained during the twelve days of Christmas. I'm pathetic.

As the saying goes, "There's no problem so bad that it can't get worse." For some reason, I was compelled to demonstrate the truth of that adage. You see, I should have felt good about losing twenty (or, er...well, ten) pounds in a year.

But I didn't.

I also should have gotten right back on the wagon. I should have kept the momentum going, putting all the Christmas cookies and the pounds and pounds of Chex Mix behind me, and tackling the problem head on.

But I didn't.

I should have looked back on the previous fifteen years of attempts and learned something from my many successes and many more failures.

But I didn't.

Keep reading. I know it's getting painful, but trust me, keep on reading.

Chapter 20

Square One

Dieters never cease to be amazed at just how true the First Law of Dieting really is. If you remember way back on page 2, this law states *weight returns at five times the velocity at which it was lost.* Time and time again, we dieters spend weeks and months losing weight only to spend days (if not hours) gaining it back.

This actually isn't as twisted as it sounds when you think about the math. Consider this scenario. What would happen to a dieter (just for the sake of argument) who reduced her caloric intake from 2,000 calories a day to zero for one week? Apart from going insane and attacking the nearest Burger King*, she'd have a total caloric deficit of 14,000 calories or four pounds. Since it's hard to eat less than zero (and discounting any additional exercise), we can conclude that this is the absolute fastest way to lose weight: four pounds per week.

Now consider the alternate scenario. Let's say this person has pancakes, syrup, sausage and orange juice for breakfast,

---

* And by that, I don't mean the restaurant, but the creepy Burger King dude himself.

a latte and two small chocolate chip muffins for a mid-morning break, burger, fries, and a Coke for lunch, a bag of chips for an afternoon snack, spaghetti & meatballs with bread and a glass of milk for dinner, and some ice cream for dessert. This clocks in at nearly 4,000 calories. Now imagine the days she drinks two sodas. Or has some cake with the ice cream. Or decides to have two bags of chips instead of one. What if it's a *really* stressful day and she has half a tub of ice cream instead of just one serving.

See? Although there's a clear lower limit to the amount of food you can eat, there's no set upper limit. Going from 2,000 calories per day to 1,600 (on a typical diet) is going to feel very slow: only 0.8 lbs per week lost. Going from 2,000 to 5,000 will move your weight along at an amazing clip: 6.0 lbs per week gained. *That's* why the weight returns so much faster than it left. Mystery solved.

The year 2006 was exceptional. Apart from proving, once again, that weight does indeed come back faster than it's lost, I set a personal record for the most Day Ones in a single year: sixteen to be exact. That works out to nearly one every three weeks for those of you still keeping score at home. It was also the first time I tried a detox diet. It was the first time I ever started a diet on Halloween. It was the first time I implemented a strict, rigorous see-food diet. And, for the first time in my life, it was the first time I actually ran out of clothes. My weight bounced up and down more than the price of gasoline. Let's take a closer look at the events just outlined.

Detox

On August 15, 2006, I began yet another grand attempt at taking control of my life. I know, I know. I'm worse than Rocky. Mickey, towel at the ready, is yelling at me from my corner, "Stay down! Stay down!" But for some insane reason, I have to get right back in there and get my head punched in for the four hundredth time. Because at this point, I was back up to 221 and ready to swear off the 220s forever. Giving up still wasn't yet an option. As always, things went well at first. I dropped maybe five pounds in ten days. But I never really felt "on" which is the first indicator that cheating is going to be very easy. And, right on schedule, there were a couple nights out where I probably shouldn't have ordered what I did. And there was at least one night in where I went a wee bit overboard on dessert. (But it was *soooo* good. I made some vanilla ice cream from scratch and then prepared cheesecake filling. These two immoral ingredients were then combined into a Super Dessert so powerful that I feared I would have to call the city for a permit to serve it.)

Fortunately, these were isolated incidents and I managed to get back to the plan for the most part. Unfortunately, after another ten days or so, things were plainly going nowhere. It seemed hard to believe I'd hit another plateau in so short a time, but there I was. So I made a decision to do something I'd never tried before: I took a diet from my diet.

After some pondering, the "detox" diet idea struck me. I don't right recall what made me think of it at the time. About all I can bring to mind now is a strong desire to clean myself up and start over.

As you may recall from page 24, the detox diet is all about getting back to basics. It's about avoiding modern and otherwise unnatural foods. (As well as disallowing certain natural items: no meat, dairy products, eggs, rice, potatoes, flour, sugar, or other white foods.) What you're left with is veggies, beans, brown rice, and other things I never, ever thought I'd eat on purpose.

So you can imagine what the Day Zero grocery shopping trip was like. Talk about a stark contrast to my low carb outings. I passed up cheese and bought carrots. I pretended not to see bacon and got broccoli instead. It was an out of body experience. Happily, it wasn't that bad. Well, except for the protein part. About the only option I had was beans, and frankly, I don't much like beans. So after wandering around the store for a while, I settled on buying hummus. I thought if I whipped up some of that and spread it over enough celery, I might be able to get by.

I also knew salads would figure prominently in this diet, so I looked for a detox-friendly dressing. If I'd known what a challenge *that* would turn out to be, I might have just signed up for Weight Watchers instead. It was nigh on impossible to find any product that didn't contain high fructose corn syrup. I was amazed at this discovery, once I actually woke up and paid attention. Sure, I could have just gone with organic dressings. They would have passed the test. But given, as a rule, that they came in four-ounce bottles costing upwards of twelve dollars a pop, I continued looking. Eventually I found most of what I needed (less the salad dressing) and I headed home, both happy and hopeful.

Day One of Fourteen. The program kicked off with the following initial stats: 220 lbs, 35% fat, 100% gross. While grocery shopping, I'd decided on soup for lunch. I found an organic, vegetable broth and decided to throw a few veggies in it. I did this without any forethought or planning and the result showed it. It was icky, icky soup. In fact, I wouldn't even go all the way to "soup." It was just nasty.

For dinner, I fixed a salad and it was worse than the soup, if that's possible. I tried making my own simple oil and vinegar dressing, but it didn't turn out well. The lettuce and the spinach weren't very good either. I think I didn't get them completely washed. A big plate of lawn clippings would have been a better meal.

To add insult to injury, about fourteen inches away was a half-eaten cheeseburger left by one of my daughters. I was so dejected and so miserable at this point that I very nearly quit right then and there. A cold, half-eaten cheeseburger would have been perfect. Only one thing got me through the wall: it was still Day One and I still wanted to give this a chance.

Day Two. There were two major advancements today. First, I went online and searched for a real soup recipe for this vegetable stock. It contained brown rice, corn, green beans, tomato sauce, spinach, and a perfect blend of spices. Oh what a difference a day can make. Second, I headed back to the store and got some real salad dressing. Lunch and dinner were indescribably better. My spirits lifted further when I reminded myself this was a two-week plan. That's it.

Day Five. By this day, I was really only eating when I felt good and ready to eat. Amazingly, I rarely felt hungry, even though I was eating far less than just the week before.

Day Seven. I came home to tacos for dinner and was very tempted to eat them. But once again, I told myself I was halfway through this and there was no reason to quit now. I had a mysterious weight gain over the weekend, but I think that was due to a small overdose of cashews.

Day Nine. My main food remained the wonderful vegetable soup (the highlight of my day), but I was starting to eat fewer veggies overall and increasing the fruit intake. Several days before, I had given up completely on the hummus. However, it didn't dawn on me until day nine that that was my only significant source of protein. That night I ditched the "no meat" rule and started adding chicken to my dinner salads. By day nine, I was down six pounds.

Day Eleven. Still going strong and down eight pounds. Woo hoo! In fact, I was so pleased with myself that I completely spaced the Fourth Law of Dieting: "Informing others of your progress immediately halts progress." Yes, I accidentally told someone I'd lost eight pounds, thus invoking the Fourth Law. And there I stayed until the end of the experiment.

Day Fifteen. Day *fifteen* of fourteen? Yes! By the time the two weeks were up, I was feeling quite right about this whole oddball experiment and decided to keep on going. I was still down "only" eight pounds, but saw no reason to quit.

Day Nineteen. As a surprise for her birthday, I flew to Chicago to see my mom. Oh no. A trip! This was the first real test of my commitment to this project. It began well. We went grocery shopping, and I bought all the things I was supposed to buy, including more spinach for my salads. I swear, the minute we got home, we heard the news about the *E. coli* outbreak and contaminated spinach. Perfect. The *one* time in my life I decide to eat veggies and they turn out bad.

The next day we met up with Jenn for lunch and went to a local deli. I scanned the menu for something that didn't look too devastating. I found it in a chicken salad sandwich.

"Do you want fries or fruit with that?" the evil, evil girl at the counter inquired.

Fries. Oh no. Fries. I *love* French fries. You all know that by now. Wild thoughts of "I've done good! I *deserve* this!" flashed through my brain when the voice of reason, perhaps for the first time in my life, prevailed.

"I'll take the fruit cup."

Whew. Disaster averted. That was a close one.

We took our numbers and found our table. After catching up for a few minutes, the waitress brought our lunches to our table. After my mom and Jenn got theirs, mine was set in front of me with a large complement of French fries.

"You ordered the fruit cup, didn't you?" Jenn asked.

"Yes, I did," vividly recalling the struggle.

"You can have them take it back," my mom offered.

"I know."

Clearly the universe wanted me to get fries. Who am I to challenge fate? The fruit cup vainly flashed through my brain, but it was too late. I could smell them. I could touch them. I was doomed.

"I've done good! I deserve this." I declared aloud to my lunch mates. "Besides, what's the worst that could happen?"

You guessed it: the kiss of death again. Will I ever learn my lesson? (Apparently not.)

Happy Halloween

Halloween is definitely one of my favorite holidays. I love that whole time of year: the cool weather, falling leaves, carving jack-o-lanterns, trick or treating, public intoxication, getting arrested, and of course eating candy. I'm not usually big on sweets. My poison is salty snacks but from time to time the sweet tooth bites me, and rarely harder than on October 31.

Getting my annual fix is like taking candy from a baby. (I knew there was a reason I had kids.) I find that the contraband I seize typically falls into two categories:

1. The stuff they don't like
2. The stuff they *do* like but will never miss.

Fortunately for them, I largely take items from the first category, such as bite sized Almond Joy bars or Hershey's Special Dark. (A *must* dipped in creamy peanut butter.) My greatest claim came just a couple years ago. Rachel, around seven or eight at the time, went up to a house, got her goods, and gleefully ran back down the driveway where I hovered, wondering what I might steal.

"Whadja get?" I called out.

"Onion rings!" she shouted back.

"Onion rings!?" I repeated in disbelief. Who would give out onion rings for Halloween? "Let me see."

I imagined her candy bucket filled with hot, greasy appetizers, fresh out of the fryer. This held promise. As it turned out, it was just a bag of Funyuns (which I seized anyway).

So you can see how starting a diet *on Halloween* would be a big deal to me. A very big deal, in fact. One has to be pretty darned fed up with oneself to not even wait one more day. And in 2006, I just happened to be that darned fed up.

What diet did I try? Who knows. Who cares. It doesn't matter. I gave it a good solid go for the better part of a week. Then on Sunday, November 5, 2006, the whole family walked Austin's *Race for the Cure*, as we do every year. It was only five kilometers but enough to get my blood pumping. This was good. It was almost like exercise. I should have taken this positive step forward and turned it into something meaningful. However, one particular item that ended up in our bag of swag was a harbinger of doom: a ten-percent off coupon to Fuddrucker's. It was there that my latest and greatest effort came to an abrupt halt. I could have ordered something healthy. I'm sure there was a chicken Caesar salad on the menu. Instead, I ate something large and greasy with a side of something fried and starchy. I enjoyed every damn bite too. It was a bit distressing afterwards, realizing that it was all over. Not just this diet, or this year, but the entire fifteen years I'd been at this lousy game.

It was all over.

The See-Food Diet

So here we are. It's November. The holidays are coming. I'm at rock bottom on so many levels. Why, I don't know about you but that sounds like the perfect recipe for an unbridled feed fest to me! Let me introduce you to the see-food diet. If you want to try your own, I highly recommend my plan. It was quite a success:

Breakfast	Eleven bowls of cereal. Six Pop-Tarts. A quart of whole milk. Pancakes and syrup for dessert.
Snack	An apple. An apple danish. Half of a one-pound bag of Doritos. A diet Coke.
Lunch	Three sausage and pepperoni Hot Pockets. French fries. Ramen noodles. Fried rice.
Snack	Two snickerdoodle cookies. The other half of the Doritos. Some Funyuns for dessert.

Dinner	A bucket of chicken planks. More French fries. Ice cream. More ice cream.
Before Bed	Eleven bowls of cereal. Six Pop-Tarts. A quart of whole milk. Pancakes and syrup for dessert.

Okay, so I'm exaggerating—a little. But this is certainly what it felt like. Nothing was off limits. Everything was fair game. And, as usual, I hated every minute of it but felt powerless to stop it.

Between the end of September and the beginning of January, less than four months all told, I went up nearly twenty-five pounds. I broke every record in my book, I believe, including a new all-time high.

This didn't quite hit home until the night of our company Christmas party. I believe I spent a solid twenty-five minutes trying on every nice shirt and pair of slacks in my closet. Nothing fit anymore. *Nothing.* Shirt after shirt came off the hangers and were thrown on the floor in disgust. Pants, too, some of which barely fit around my ankles. I was driven mad with utter disbelief. "Are these actually my clothes? Did I ever actually fit into these!?"

Just as I was about to give up and wear a sweat suit to the party, I found one last pair of pants in the furthest reaches of the closet. It was a Christmas miracle: *they fit.* Not perfectly, of course, but I could definitely get them buttoned, which is more than I could say for the previous eight attempts. I quickly searched for the least-problematic shirt on the floor and threw on a jacket, itself unbuttonable, but serviceable. It would be enough to get me by for the evening.

I made it through the party trying not to breathe too much. And as miserable as I was, I *still* ate too much, even going so far as to visit the dessert table. (Clearly, clearly out of my mind. Either that or just resigned to the fact that I was destined to be the subject of a show on *The Learning Channel* someday.)

The good news is we didn't stay long. Dying to get out of these clothes, I drove home at roughly 132 MPH. A cop stopped me but when I explained the issue, he not only let me go, but gave me an escort home. So it was with no little relief that I peeled the clothes off the second I got home and replaced them with the aforementioned sweats. "Ahhh! I could live in these forever." (Hmmm...maybe I shouldn't speak any words of ill omen. It may come to that yet.)

Just FYI, all those discarded shirts and pants are, in fact, still on my closet floor right now: a daily reminder that I still have a lot of work ahead of me.

So here we have the wonderful year 2006 in review:

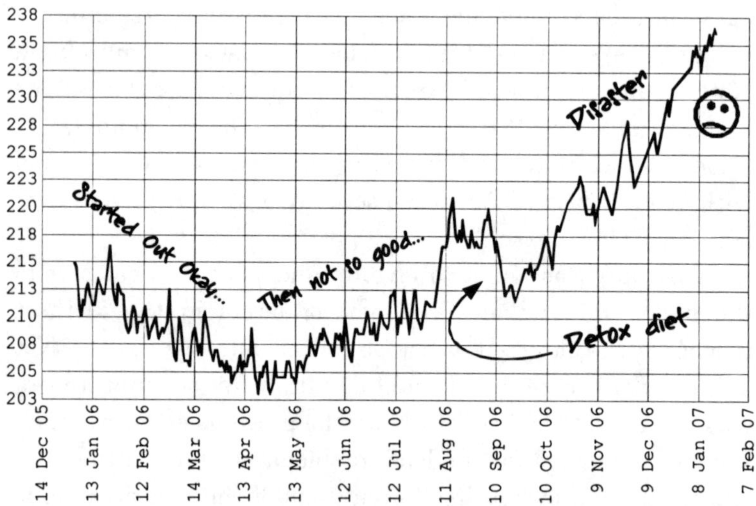

And he lived miserably ever after.

Chapter 21

Ever After

Hitting an all-time high was the worst. Sure, I'd been steadily gaining it all back for six years. I saw it coming from miles and miles away. Yet, at the same time, I *didn't* see it coming. Therapists have a technical term for that: denial.

So where does one go from here? At some point, doesn't one just finally accept one's fate? How many attempts? How many failures? How many times must a man try to lose weight, before you can call him a loser? The answer, my friend, is...well, if it *is* blowin' in the wind, then maybe we should ask Bob Dylan for it.

I wish I had the answer, but I don't. If you just read two hundred pages hoping to find it then I owe you an apology.* Maybe the answer will *always* be blowing in the wind, just outside our grasp. Or maybe it's just around the corner. The Magic Pill might come out next month. Scientists may discover the Fat Gene and blast us with gamma rays to alter our DNA. We'll be thin again Real Soon Now. Just pass me that box of Cheez-Its while I wait.

---

* Tell you what, I'll buy you a Happy Meal and we'll call it even.

Your last diet failed you for a million reasons. I've covered a few of the causes in this book. I've missed many more. But enough with the fluff. Let's finally get to the important part of this book.

How This Book Won't Help You on Your Next Diet

One afternoon back in college, as I walked between classes, I stopped outside a professor's office. Among the cartoons and assorted clippings taped to the door was a list entitled, "The Laws of Project Management." They were all very funny (and true) but one that stood out among the rest stated, "No project has ever been completed on time, within budget, or with the same people that started it. Yours will not be the first."

I hope by now you realize how this book won't help you on your next diet. If not, then I've spent too much time goofing off and not enough time getting to the point. Luckily, it's a simple point, so if I have missed it I can easily squeeze it in now. No diet book has ever solved the diet problem. Mine will not be the first.

Diet books can give you advice and ideas. Diet foods can help you cut calories and eat better. Diet groups can give you encouragement and support. But nothing—and by that I mean *nothing*—can make you lose weight but *you*. True success comes from the inside and none of my stories or jokes or facts or fiction will change that. Not this book, not the million that came before it, nor the million that will certainly follow. Open your eyes and look around. The evidence is everywhere.

It's simply time for you to give up hope. Give up hope that the pill is coming. Give up hope that the next fad diet will be *the one*. Give up hope that calorie-free corn chips and queso dip are just around the corner.

But don't give up hope in yourself. Realize that you and you alone will be the one to figure this out and make it work. It's okay to have outside help. Just don't expect the outside help to do it all for you. If you're not ready on the inside, then all the diet gurus in the world could come and live with you for a year and it wouldn't matter.

So how do you get there? How do you "flip the switch" and make a real, permanent commitment to get where you want to be? To be honest, I have no idea. If I had the answer to that, I'd write a book. All I can offer is encouragement; I can't offer a blueprint. That said, I might have inadvertently (even presciently) put it best when I wrote a note to myself on January 2, 2005:

> I don't need a plan. I don't need a miracle. I need a decision. I need to decide to make a difference, and nothing in the world can give that to me. I must give it to myself. Once that's done, the rest will follow. It won't be easy.

So there you go. That's what I offer you. If you turn this into something, don't give me an ounce of credit, because *you* did it all. That's exactly why this book won't help you on your next diet.

How This Book May Help Others

The diet industry takes in an absolutely astounding amount of money. I've read figures ranging from eighteen to thirty five *billion* dollars or more per year in the United States alone. You heard right, people are spending upwards of one hundred million dollars per day for one reason: they just want to be smaller. They spend money on diet foods and diet programs and diet surgeries. They spend money on supplements and herbs and magic pills. They buy books and magazines and videos. They join health clubs and purchase equipment for home. One hundred million dollars per day and all we have to show for it is endless news reports all saying the same thing: we're getting larger and larger and larger, and there's no end in sight.

When confronted with that thirty-five billion dollar figure, many people are appalled that such an obscene amount of money changes hands each year. The next reaction is predictable: "All they have to do is eat less and exercise! There's no reason to spend that much money on such a simple problem with an obvious solution."

I won't even bother to respond to that statement. That's what the rest of this book is all about.

What slightly fewer people pick up on is the raw, dark irony of the total picture. By some estimates, thirty-eight million people in the United States are "food insecure," meaning they cannot sustain minimum food needs due to a lack of money. And almost a third of those are truly hungry and malnourished. This country is wealthy enough to feed itself many times over, yet millions go without. An extremely overweight population is a growing concern at all levels, yet hunger is on the rise. In one household, a woman will spend $100 on diet pills while only a few miles away another woman is unable to put food on her table. Something is seriously wrong with this picture.

The causes are many and complex. No two situations are identical and therefore, no single solution exists. It may be that there *is* no solution. We may have already passed the point where a problem can become so large, difficult, and involved that it truly is unsolvable. But that in no way means we shouldn't try. If you can't feed one thousand people, try to feed one hundred. If you can't do that, then try fifty, ten, or even one. Something is definitely better than nothing.

The magnitude of the issue is mind-boggling. It's difficult to consider that for each hungry person in this country roughly $1,000 is spent on weight loss every year. Wouldn't it be nice if some of that money went to where it's needed? Now I'm not suggesting in any way that the diet industry turn over every cent to fight hunger. We have about three or four more visits from Haley's Comet before that happens. But something is definitely better than nothing. What's wrong with starting out small?

While this isn't my first book, it *is* the first one that has the potential of reaching an audience greater than two dozen readers. As I tap out these words on my keyboard, late at night, slouched in my chair at my under-lit desk, I have no idea what will happen. It may never sell a single copy. It might be a best-seller. Who knows? All I can say for sure is that on the one-in-a-billion chance this book actually *does* do well on the market, I'd like to steer a good deal of those profits towards people who can't get food.

How much? I don't rightly know. If this book sells one hundred copies, I will keep the twelve dollars in profit and buy myself a new office chair at a garage sale. If it sells one thousand copies, I might be able to afford one or two college textbooks for my kids. But if for some strange reason it outsells Atkins, South Beach, and Dr. Phil combined, then I just might be able to help out a few people in the process. I can't give an exact figure. For the lowly, unknown author like me, that point is so far away it can't even be seen with the naked eye. I only promise this: the greater the sales, the greater the percentage. I'll keep you posted.

Me, I'm still hanging in there. Like so many times before, I got myself back on track on Monday. And, just like so many times before, I've lost two or three pounds already. I'm eating a little less and walking a little more, and can't complain. There's a lot to be said for small moves.

Today is Friday. Most normal people live for Fridays, but I'm not normal people. I think time flies fast enough without wishing for weekends to hurry up and arrive. For that reason, I find that Fridays do little more than serve as a reminder of two panic-inducing thoughts:

1. Time is fleeting.
2. The previous six days were very unproductive.

But today is different because I'm doing something I never thought I'd actually do. I'm writing the final two pages of this book. So on this particular Friday, I'm not feeling quite as unproductive as I usually do. In fact, I actually feel pretty good and there's a lot to be said for that too. Of course, Friday also means one other thing: pizza night. But don't worry! This latest diet has produced some results. I've resisted worse temptations than this. In fact, just last week at work someone came by my office and...

Oh. Hang on a sec. There's the doorbell. I'll be right back.

Okay, I'm back. It was the pizza delivery guy. He brought two this time: one pepperoni on thin crust and the other plain cheese for the kids. I took it to the kitchen, called the troops in, and started to fix myself a small chicken Caesar salad.

It sure smells good though. And you all know how much I love the pepperoni. But no! I'm on a diet. It's going well and I see no reason to mess that up. Temptations are temporary but pizza is permanent.

But I did mention how good it smelled, didn't I? I mean, I've done good. I deserve this. Just a couple bites won't hurt. Or maybe even a slice or two (or six).

Besides, what's the worst that could happen?